ALLEN CARR
With John Dicey

EASY WAY
TO QUIT
CANNABIS

ALLEN CARR

With John Dicey

EASY WAY
TO QUIT
CANNABIS

Dedication

To Cris Hay, who is not only a highly accomplished 'Top Gun' Allen Carr's Easyway Therapist (whose work has spanned three decades), but also possesses a brilliant mind which has been brought to bear with dedication, finesse and potency to help apply the method to a wide variety of addictions and issues. A key member of the team and a great friend.

Also to the brilliant Tim Glynne-Jones and Tania O'Donnell for their great skill, good humour and invaluable assistance in making this book happen.

ARCTURUS

This edition published in 2022 by Arcturus Publishing Limited
26/27 Bickels Yard, 151–153 Bermondsey Street,
London SE1 3HA, UK

ISBN: 978-1-3988-0518-7
AD008673UK

Printed in the UK

MIX
Paper from
responsible sources
FSC® C018072

Allen Carr

Allen Carr was a chain-smoker for over 30 years. In 1983, after countless failed attempts to quit, he went from 60–100 cigarettes a day to zero without suffering withdrawal pangs, without using willpower, and without putting on weight. He realised that he had discovered what the world had been waiting for – the easy way to stop smoking – and embarked on a mission to help cure the world's smokers.

As a result of the phenomenal success of his method, he gained an international reputation as the world's leading expert on stopping smoking and his network of centres now spans the globe. His first book, Allen Carr's Easy Way to Stop Smoking, has sold over 17 million copies, remains a global bestseller, and has been published in more than 40 different languages. Hundreds of thousands of smokers have successfully quit at Allen Carr's Easyway centres where, with a success rate of over 90 per cent, it's guaranteed you'll find it easy to stop or your money back.

Allen Carr's brilliant Easyway method has been successfully applied to weight control, alcohol, debt, refined sugar, cocaine, cannabis, and a host of other addictions and issues.

For more information about Allen Carr's Easyway, please visit **www.allencarr.com**

ALLEN CARR'S EASYWAY

The key that will set you free

CONTENTS

CONTENTS

It's important that you don't skip this important

Introduction

by John Dicey, Global CEO and Senior Therapist, Allen Carr's Easyway

Welcome to *Allen Carr's Easy Way to Quit Cannabis*. Allen Carr's reputation in the field of addiction treatment was built on his huge success in helping smokers to quit. His Easyway method was so successful that it quickly became, and remains, a global phenomenon. From the earliest days of Easyway, Allen was inundated with requests from sufferers of countless other addictions and issues, imploring him to relate his method to their drug or issue. By the turn of the century, Allen had assembled a team of bright, loyal and dedicated senior therapists who went on to help him not only apply the method to all those addictions and issues but to play a key role in delivering Allen Carr's Easyway method across the globe.

The responsibility for ensuring our books are faithful to Allen Carr's original method is mine and it's an honour to be writing this important introduction. Rest assured, once you've read it, I'll leave you in Allen's capable hands.

It has been suggested to me that I describe myself as the author of the books we've published since Allen passed away. In my view, that would be quite wrong.

That's because every new book is written strictly in accordance with Allen Carr's brilliant Easyway method. In our new books, we have merely updated the content, context, and format to make them as relevant as possible for the modern-day audience, whilst also incorporating upgraded elements of the method developed during the tens of thousands of hours spent treating addicts of all kinds at our live seminars. There is not a word in our books that Allen didn't write or wouldn't have written if he was still with us and, for that reason, the updates, anecdotes and analogies that are not his own work – that were contemporised or added by me – are written clearly in Allen's voice to seamlessly complement the original text and method.

I consider myself privileged to have worked very closely with Allen on Easyway books while he was still alive, gaining insight into how the method could be applied, and we explored and mapped out its future evolution together. I was more than happy to have the responsibility for continuing this vital mission placed on my shoulders by Allen himself. It's a responsibility I accepted with humility and one I take extremely seriously.

WHAT ARE OUR CREDENTIALS?

We've been treating addicts all over the world with phenomenal success over the past 35 years. The senior members of my team and I were inspired to join Allen's quest for one simple reason: his method saved our lives. Like every Allen Carr's Easyway Therapist in the world, we were drawn to get involved in Easyway as a result of being set free from our own addictions.

It was a pleasure to work with Allen in assembling the most remarkable senior therapist team to set about the task of applying the method to issues other than smoking, so that it could help people escape from the misery of alcohol addiction, weight issues, sugar addiction, as well as cocaine, cannabis and opioid addiction and a host of other addictions and issues.

The drug-taking history of Allen's senior therapist team, far from deterring Allen and myself from recruiting them, encouraged us to do so. If Allen was impressed by your drive, enthusiasm, ability and accomplishments, he considered it a superb bonus if you had previously experienced the misery of other addictions. He was acutely aware that it would be extremely difficult to apply his method to the full range of addictions without the direct involvement of people who had used the method to set themselves free from those drugs. Whether it be heroin, cocaine, cannabis, alcohol, nicotine, serious weight issues or sugar addiction, direct, up-close-and-personal experience of those drugs and issues enabled Allen and his team to develop the method accordingly.

This book is the direct result of our experience in treating cannabis addicts for more than 20 years at Allen Carr's flagship centre in London. Addicts have flown in from every corner of the globe to seek our help. So, rest assured, this program is tried-and-tested, and is effective regardless of your nationality or location. When we started treating cannabis addiction, we were so confident in the programme we had created that we even provided the same money-back guarantee for cannabis addicts that we had been providing to smokers since the inception of the method. If they didn't quit the drug, we refunded their fee in full. The treatment is expensive – for cannabis, and other drugs, the live seminars are delivered on a one-to-one basis, as opposed to our other seminars which are normally delivered in groups of 20-25 people – so, naturally, we have to charge more. But we were determined to ensure that people buying the service could do so with absolute confidence. If they completed the programme and failed to quit the drug, their fee was refunded in full.

Over the past 20 years, in spite of the relative expense of the live one-to-one cannabis seminars, the refund rate has been less than 5% and we continue to offer the money-back guarantee to this day (and the live seminars delivered via Zoom are equally effective). There are a whole host of eye-wateringly expensive rehab treatment centres around the world, yet we remain, to our knowledge, the only provider of addiction services that provides any form of money-back guarantee. How can we do that?

SIMPLE: THIS METHOD WORKS!

Our motivation for putting the method down in writing and into an online video programme was to enable anyone, anywhere in the world, regardless of their level of wealth, to benefit from *Allen Carr's Easy Way to Quit Cannabis*. This book isn't simply a transcript of our live one-to-one Seminars – those are dynamic, interactive, last six hours, include telephone/email support and free-of-charge back-up sessions – but, like our Online Video Programme, it is certainly the next best thing.

Make no mistake, this book is a complete programme in itself so please don't be put off by the mention of the live seminars or the online video programme. You have in your hands the most up-to-date, cutting-edge version of Allen Carr's Easyway to Quit Cannabis method and this book will set you free.

Cannabis is consumed in many forms: weed, hash, skunk, smoked neat or mixed with tobacco, vaped, through a bong, eaten, the list goes on. For the sake of simplicity, throughout this book we refer to it simply as cannabis, dope or a joint. Please take that to mean your cannabis consumption, however you take it.

I'm aware that many people who are unfamiliar with the method, or who have never met people who have successfully quit with Easyway, assume that some of the claims made about it are far-fetched or exaggerated. That was certainly my reaction when I first heard them. I was incredibly fortunate to have had my life saved by Allen Carr. There is no doubt that had I not come into contact with Allen and his amazing method, more than a little reluctantly I should add, in the late 1990s I wouldn't have made it to the 21st century. I was so inspired by my new-found freedom I couldn't wait to offer Allen my assistance to help him achieve his goals.

I'm incredibly proud to have headed up the team which, over the past 23 years, has taken Allen's method from Berlin to Brasília, from New Zealand to New York, from Sydney to Santiago and beyond.

I still take pleasure in deflecting all the praise and acclaim straight back to the great man himself: it's all down to Allen Carr.

The method is as pure, as bright, as adaptable and as effective as it's ever been, allowing us to apply it to a whole host of addictions and issues. Whether it's cannabis, cocaine, heroin, alcohol or sugar addiction, gambling or junk spending, fear of flying, mindfulness, or even digital/social media addiction, the method guides those who need help in a simple, relatable, plain-speaking way.

Please don't mistake Allen Carr's Easyway method for some kind of 'Jack of all trades', as you're about to discover for yourself, there is no doubt that it truly is, the master of all addictions.

Now, without further delay, let me pass you into the safest of hands – Allen Carr and his 'Easyway'.

Chapter 1

THE KEY

Congratulations on reaching this important stage in your bid to be free from cannabis. You may think you're right at the beginning but you're actually very close to success already.

By choosing to read this book (and it *is* your choice), you have taken the most important step anyone can take in conquering addiction. It is a step in the right direction – a step away from the misconceptions that keep cannabis users trapped in a cycle of addiction and a step towards the truth: that quitting for good can be easy, provided you follow the right method.

This method has been proven to work, time after time after time. All the information you need to follow the method and set yourself free is contained in this book. Not only will you be free, you will stay free and you will find it ridiculously easy. That's the whole point of Easyway.

At this stage you may well find that a little hard to believe. No-one finds it easy to quit, do they? Well, yes they do – millions of people, in fact. But don't worry if you feel a little sceptical right now. It's important that you question everything, because that will make it easier for you to see the truth. The reason people find it hard to quit is because they're brainwashed with lies and myths and illusions.

You might be surprised to learn that virtually everything you think you know about cannabis is actually the opposite of the truth. Hold that thought. We'll return to it later.

A METHOD THAT WORKS

I discovered this method while trying to quit smoking. For more than 30 years I chain-smoked 60-100 cigarettes a day. I had tried all the conventional methods to quit, including willpower, nicotine replacement, all kinds of substitutes and gimmicks, but nothing worked.

It was like being caught between the devil and the deep blue sea. I desperately wanted to quit but whenever I tried, I was utterly miserable. No matter how long I survived I never felt completely free – it was as if I'd lost my best friend, my crutch, my character, my very personality. In those days I really believed that there were such types as addictive personalities or that there was something in our genes that meant we couldn't enjoy life or cope with stress without the drug.

Sound familiar?

Eventually, after countless failed attempts, I gave up even trying to stop and resigned myself to a lifetime of slavery and an early death. Then I discovered something that motivated me to try again.

I went overnight from a hundred cigarettes a day to zero, without any bad temper or sense of loss, void, or depression. On the contrary, I actually enjoyed the process.

It didn't take me long to realise that I had discovered a method that could enable any smoker to quit, easily, immediately, without feeling deprived, without using willpower, substitutes, or other gimmicks, without suffering depression or unpleasant withdrawal symptoms and without gaining weight.

After trying out the method on friends and relatives with great success, I gave up my successful career in the financial world to devote myself to helping other smokers quit. I called the method Easyway and it has become a global success, with centres in over 150 cities in more than 50 countries worldwide. Bestselling books based on my method are now translated into more than 40 languages, with more being added each year.

So what's this got to do with your cannabis addiction? Quitting smoking is one thing but "getting off drugs"… that's a whole different kettle of fish isn't it?

Nicotine happens to be one of the most addictive drugs on the planet. And I soon realised that my method could be applied successfully to any drug addiction. And so it proved. Easyway has helped tens of millions of people quit smoking, alcohol, cocaine, cannabis, opioids, sugar addiction and achieve freedom from weight issues, junk-spending, gambling addiction, caffeine addiction, fear of flying, and even tech addiction for those who have issues with smartphones, gaming and digital overload.

You've heard the expression 'Jack of all trades, master of none.' Well, when it came to conquering addictions, Easyway mastered them all. Including cannabis.

HOW IT WORKS

Easyway works by removing the sense of deprivation that addicts suffer when they try to quit with other methods. It removes the feeling that you are making a sacrifice. Unlike other methods you may have tried, it does not rely on willpower.

All you have to do is read this book to the end, follow all of the instructions and you will be set free from your addiction to cannabis.

Some cannabis users balk at the word 'addiction'. Compared to other drugs, cannabis tends to be regarded as being quite benign, harmless, almost not worth worrying about. It actually doesn't matter whether you consider yourself an addict, or just someone who has a little too much, a little too often, the fact is you're looking for a way out and this method works for anyone who wants to stop using cannabis.

So don't get bogged down with the label 'addict'. But don't reject it either. The great news is that you're all set to put the entire issue behind you. If you don't see yourself as an addict, you obviously do regard yourself as someone who uses cannabis and wishes you didn't. That's who this book is for. It's going to set you free, so don't let any quibbles over terminology get in the way.

QUITTING WITHOUT WILLPOWER

Most addicts are convinced that quitting is difficult. First you have to overcome the physical withdrawal and then there's the craving.

The good news is that with this method, you will discover that withdrawal 'pains' are so minuscule you barely notice them and once you've quit there is no craving, so there is absolutely no need for willpower, or even substitutes to 'ease you off'.

You won't suffer that feeling of deprivation either because you won't be 'giving up' anything. There is no sacrifice. Instead you will be enjoying a better life, free from slavery. If you have tried to quit cannabis in the past and failed, if you have battled against feelings of deprivation and sacrifice and ended up succumbing to temptation, please put those experiences behind you.

THIS METHOD IS DIFFERENT.

This time you're going to approach quitting from an entirely different angle. You won't be brow-beaten about the downsides of the addiction: the physical harm, the cost, the slavery, the shame, the low self-esteem, the feelings of hopelessness, weakness, of not being 'you' any more, the destruction of relationships, the feelings of isolation, of not fulfilling your potential.

That would be patronising and pointless.

If those factors were going to help you get free from your addiction, they would have done so by now and you wouldn't be reading this book. Rather than trying to use those downsides to scare you into quitting, this method requires you to ignore them. Once you're free, release from them simply becomes a wonderful bonus.

Instead, think about this question:

WHAT'S SO GREAT ABOUT BEING A CANNABIS ADDICT?

We'll return to that later.

For now, rest assured, you're on a well-trodden path. More than 50 million people have used my Easyway method. They didn't come across the method as a result of lavish marketing and advertising campaigns, they discovered it via the oldest and most reliable means of referral: word of mouth.

The best advertisement for Easyway has always been the people who have used it to quit. They are so delighted, they just want to sing its praises. We don't have to ask them to do so. And of course their family, friends and colleagues see the evidence with their own eyes.

They see that their loved ones are not suffering, they're not hiding away, fearful that they might fall back into addiction. In fact, they simply appear to have carried on enjoying life, handling stress, relaxing, socialising and having fun, coping with the ups and downs of life without showing the slightest interest in taking the drug again. It doesn't matter whether it's nicotine, alcohol, cannabis, cocaine, sugar or any other drug; the effect is always the same:

UNBRIDLED FREEDOM.

WHY YOU'RE READING THIS BOOK

It was literally word of mouth that carried news of my method across the globe in those early days, well before the birth of the internet, social media and digital marketing. It became a global phenomenon at breakneck speed the old-fashioned way.

Of course, more recently, word of mouth has become even speedier and more effective. With social media, bloggers and instant communication, good news travels faster than ever.

In fact, it's quite likely that the reason you're reading this book – the means by which you originally discovered Easyway – was via a member of your family, a friend or a colleague telling you of their own success with the method.

Now it's your turn. Get set to be free from cannabis.

This is the first day of an exciting adventure: the day you start preparing yourself to be free. All you need to do is follow the instructions.

Your first instruction is:

FOLLOW ALL OF THE INSTRUCTIONS.

That is the key. And as long as you stick to it, it will release you.

Think of it as the combination to a safe. You could spend a lifetime trying to break into the safe and never succeed. But if you know the correct combination, it's ridiculously easy. Miss out just one number in the combination or lose the key and the safe that holds your freedom within it stays locked.

This book contains the key: the combination of information you need in order to become free. It will enable you to escape from your cannabis addiction. Follow the instructions and you will succeed. Ignore any one of them and you jeopardise your entire objective.

Your second instruction is:

DON'T ATTEMPT TO CUT DOWN.

It's important that you don't try to control your cannabis use until you are advised to do so. That will be towards the end of this book.

If, however, you have already abstained for a few days, there is no need to carry on using it. But if you decide to read this book over the next few days and tonight you're out with friends or at home and want to have a joint, do so. I don't want you using willpower to resist your desire for a smoke because that would interfere with the method.

But be sure to only read this book when you are not under the influence of any drug, including alcohol.

Chapter 2

THINK POSITIVELY

To find it easy to quit you must achieve a positive frame of mind; one whereby whenever you think about cannabis you feel a sense of release, freedom and relief that you don't use it anymore. That really is the only way to become, and remain, truly free and no longer vulnerable to the drug.

Correcting your perception of cannabis in this way will be an exciting, eye-opening and positive experience. You might find that hard to believe but you have absolutely nothing to lose and everything to gain by accepting that it's going to be exactly that way.

Your third instruction is:

START OFF IN A HAPPY FRAME OF MIND.

Closely followed by the fourth instruction:

THINK POSITIVELY.

Push aside any feelings of impending doom and gloom. Nothing bad is going to happen and there is no need to be miserable or anticipate failure or difficulty. You're about to achieve something truly wonderful, something amazing.

Regard your short journey through this programme as it really is: an exciting challenge, an adventure. Just think how proud you will feel when you're free. This might be a private achievement for you, something that will remain a secret from those who are nearest and dearest to you, but don't let that temper the feeling of pride. You are about to impress the most important person on the planet:

YOU!

The fifth instruction is the most difficult to follow:

KEEP AN OPEN MIND.

The importance of this cannot be overemphasised. Some people believe that Easyway is itself a form of brainwashing. In a way, that's a tribute to its effectiveness but, in fact, nothing could be further from the truth.

This method is all about:

COUNTER-BRAINWASHING.

If you imagine brainwashing as the gradual, damaging over-tightening of a coil or spring... all we do, over the course of a few hours, is gradually, painlessly and safely, stop the unnatural and damaging over-tightening process and then gently and calmly reverse it, eventually leaving the coil or spring in its natural, healthy, safe condition. That's counter-brainwashing.

This method involves the reversal of false beliefs that you may have had your entire life. You need to question what you think you know about cannabis. Question what society, other addicts and even your own experiences have led you to believe about the drug. If you can do that and you follow all the other instructions, you cannot fail.

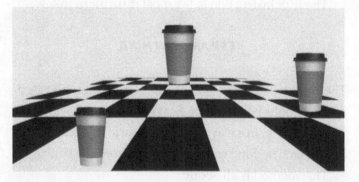

Take a look at these different sized coffee cups. If someone told you they're all the same size you would question their judgement, wouldn't you? You've already accepted that they're different sizes because that's what I told you and that's what you see.

Nevertheless, the fact is, they're all exactly the same size.

Look again. Still sceptical? Take a ruler and measure them. Surprising, isn't it?

The reason for showing you this illusion is to demonstrate how the mind can be easily tricked into accepting something as true when, in fact, it's entirely false.

Your only frame of reference regarding cannabis is your addicted state of mind and body. In that context, a spliff does seem to deliver a boost. In reality, though, it's dragging you down, mentally and physically.

WHO'S IN CONTROL?

Do you believe that you take cannabis out of choice? That's the general assumption. After all, no-one's holding a gun to your head. You're the one who buys it and you're the one who takes it. But are you really acting out of free will?

Compare it to a financial investment that backfires. You see a friend appearing to get good returns so you're tempted to join them and invest yourself. But it turns out that the investment is a confidence trick, which results in you and your friend losing your money. Would you hold your hands up and say you had made a genuine choice?

If you invest in something based on phoney information, and continue to invest even though you're losing your money, you haven't chosen to lose your money, you've been conned.

This is a crucial point. It's not the case that you made a poorly judged investment; the fact is you never stood a chance. It was a con. A rip-off.

Your cannabis use is the result of a similar con trick. You made the decision to start using it, but that decision was based on flawed information. You continued to use it based on a combination of the same misinformation and addiction.

Of course you chose to have those first experimental joints, but how long ago was that? Years ago? Perhaps you were at an entirely different stage of your life? You were excited. It felt illicit. It felt sophisticated. It felt dangerous. But at no point in those early days did you decide to end up in your current predicament, having been dragged down so low by the drug that you had to seek professional help to stop taking it.

You're not reading this book because cannabis has become a slight inconvenience to you, nor because it occurred to you that it might be nice to stop taking it. You chose to read this book because at some point, perhaps some time ago, you suddenly realised:

YOU'RE TRAPPED.

Yes, it was your decision to start using cannabis but at some imperceptible stage you realised the reverse had became true: cannabis was using you.

In all honesty, you knew this fairly early on but you brushed the thought aside. After all, you were convinced that you could take it or leave it – or at least that if you really wanted to stop taking it you could.

At what point did you decide that you would need to take cannabis several times a month. Or every week? Or more days than not? Or even every day? At what point did you decide that, even if you didn't take it every day then you would end up bingeing on it, sometimes for days in a row, never being allowed to stop, just delaying and holding out for as long as possible until the next time and the next time and the next time?

You didn't decide to become a cannabis addict and you didn't decide that you would need to take it for the rest of your life. The simple truth is:

YOU DON'T CONTROL THE DRUG –
THE DRUG CONTROLS YOU.

You know deep down that it controls you. And you know what it's cost you, not only financially. You no longer use cannabis because it feels exciting, In fact, you're probably bored with it. You no longer take it because it feels cool. In fact, it makes you feel anything but cool, doesn't it? And you don't take it because it's illicit or dangerous. You take it in spite of that.

WHY YOU WANT TO QUIT

Clients who attend our one-to-one live seminars for cannabis addiction give a variety of reasons why they want to quit.

"I want to feel in control again."

"I'm scared about losing my partner... my family... my job."

"I've finally acknowledged that I've got a problem."

"I'm addicted."

"I'm worried about the money and how it tires me out."

"It's causing me health problems."

"It's separating me from my family and friends."

"I know I'm a better person than this."

"Life is getting bad – I feel a bit hollow and empty."

"It's destroying my relationships."

"The effect that it's having on my body – but also on my mind."

"It's ruining my social relationships."

"Health, money, family."

"I thought it would help with my depression but it's just made it worse."

"It has taken over my life and I've finally had enough."

"I'm out of control, I feel bored and unmotivated and it's affecting my work."

"It's taking over my life, making me depressed."

No doubt you can relate to at least some of these factors, maybe even all of them, as well as some others that I haven't mentioned.

If you feel at all resistant to the idea that you no longer take cannabis out of choice, you need to ask yourself why you chose to read this book. If you are in control of your drug use, exercising free will, why not just choose not to take it anymore?

It's not quite as simple as that, is it? Here's why:

Because you're an addict.

CUTTING DOWN

How many times have you tried to quit cannabis? Or just cut down? You get by for a few days, or a week, or even a month or even more, but eventually you get sucked back in. And this time it always seems harder to resist, doesn't it? You want it more frequently, earlier in the week, earlier in the day. Just more.

The fact is that cutting down and trying to control or limit the intake of a drug to which you're addicted simply does not work. Telling someone to limit their intake of an addictive drug is like telling them they can jump off a building as long as they don't fall more than a few metres. The force of addiction, just like the force of gravity, will always drag you down. Yet many so-called experts still prescribe cutting down. Ignore them.

Later in the book we will explain why your previous attempts to quit might have ended with you falling back even deeper into the trap. More importantly, you will develop a clear understanding as to why this time will be different and why you'll not only get free but stay free.

Having acknowledged that the reason you take cannabis isn't because you want to, or choose to, but simply because you're addicted to it, here is some fabulous news:

THE ADDICTION IS ACTUALLY EASY TO BREAK. JUST AS LONG AS YOU KNOW HOW.

Chapter 3

THE TRAP

It can be frightening to admit that you're addicted to a drug. That word "addiction" is one we associate with hard drug users, like heroin addicts. The good news is that your addiction to cannabis is easy to break. In fact, all addictions are much easier to break than we are led to believe. It's just a question of understanding how the addiction works.

Once you can see that, it becomes equally clear what you need to do to get free.

Cannabis is a physically addictive drug, which means that after you consume it, it creates physical withdrawal. This is a mild, empty, slightly insecure, slightly uptight feeling – so mild, in fact, that it's almost imperceptible.

When you take your next dose of the drug, that mild, empty, insecure feeling temporarily disappears, leaving you feeling normal again. In fact, you take each dose of cannabis merely to try to return to the feeling you had all the time before you became addicted. That said, it's such a gradual process, you're not even aware that it's happening.

Think of it as a little monster inside your body that feeds on dope. If you don't feed it, it complains. Feed it and the complaining stops for a while, only to return as your body withdraws again from the latest dose. When you break free from the addiction, you're going to starve that Little Monster to death.

This won't be hard. The physical withdrawal is very slight, remember. You go through it whenever you're not taking cannabis. People go days and sometimes weeks without responding to it. Getting rid of the Little Monster is no more daunting than living with those almost imperceptible complaints for a little while. It's easy provided you're in the right frame of mind and follow some simple instructions.

What makes quitting difficult for people who follow the wrong method is not the Little Monster – physical withdrawal itself – but the fact that it acts as a trigger for the real problem:

THE BIG MONSTER.

The Little Monster is created the first time you take cannabis. The Big Monster is created by brainwashing, and actually exists in most of us, whether or not we ever take drugs of any sort.

Even from an early age, we are brainwashed – often by people trying to put us off ever taking drugs – into believing that there is some kind of benefit or crutch to be had from cannabis. It's widely publicised that it helps us to relax, or feel calm, or feel a sense of release or abandon. We're told it helps us handle stress and pressure, and aspects of life that we don't necessarily want to confront. Some people even think they can't concentrate, focus or be creative without the drug. The small distractions of the Little Monster seems to confirm this.

When you take the drug, that empty, insecure, slightly uptight feeling that it created disappears for a while and you do feel less empty, less insecure and less uptight than a moment before. Withdrawal makes you feel physically lethargic whilst mentally restless. It is distracting and, therefore, does impair concentration.

Each puff seems to relieve these symptoms and we are fooled into believing that we get a genuine pleasure or crutch from it. It's this belief that creates the feeling of deprivation when we try to quit. And it's this feeling of deprivation which creates the strong cravings associated with cannabis withdrawal.

Remember, the physical withdrawal (the Little Monster) is very mild. It's the thought process that it triggers, aided and abetted by the brainwashing (the Big Monster), that causes the unpleasant cravings.

This method eradicates the Big Monster. All you have to do then is starve the Little Monster to death by stopping taking the drug.

THE PITCHER PLANT

The progress of addiction is so slight, it happens without us really noticing. It's a subtle process that traps its victims in much the same way as a pitcher plant.

A pitcher plant is a carnivorous plant, shaped like a pitcher, with a tall, slender, jug-like body that opens up to a wider rim. The scent of its nectar attracts flies, which land on the rim and sip the nectar. The slope at the top is so gradual that the fly doesn't realise that it is being gradually lured further into the pitcher. By the time the slope has become steeper, the fly is too preoccupied with the nectar to notice.

When it gets beyond the neck of the vase, the fly can see many dead insects in a pool of liquid at the bottom. But that doesn't bother it, as it knows it can fly away whenever it likes. So it feels quite safe continuing to gorge on the nectar. By the time it's had enough and decides to fly off, it is too far in to do so.

The fly panics and begins to struggle, but the more it struggles to escape, the more it covers itself in the sticky nectar, which weighs it down even more and makes it

for it to get a grip on the sides of the plant,
ow vertical.

y the fly ends up joining the other dead insects
ive juice and the bottom of the pitcher.

point would you say the fly lost control?

slid into the digestive juice? When it tried to
ound it couldn't? No, that was when it *realised*

it   ontrol, so it must have been before then.

hen it saw all the dead insects at the bottom
of tl   ? Or was it somewhere on the gradual slope
at the

Many people will maintain that the fly was in control
at both those stages, because it could have escaped if it
had wanted to. But it didn't choose to escape at either
of those points. Why? Because it didn't realise it was in
a trap.

So when did the fly lose control?

Was it when it first landed on the lip of the plant? No,
it was even before that.

THE FLY WAS NEVER IN CONTROL.

It was subtly being controlled by the plant from the
moment it got a whiff of the nectar.

That perfectly describes how we become victims
to the myth of dope before we even take it. We become

hooked without even realising it. The brainwashing, the reputation and perceived advantages of the drug are all around us, in movies and literature, amongst our friends and peers. As soon as we first try it, it seems to confirm the brainwashing. And that's when we lose control.

Of course, we know we're not really in control quite early on, but we push it to the back of our minds. We think we could easily escape if we wanted to.

The good news is that, unlike the fly, you're not standing on a slippery slope; there is no physical force compelling you to take more cannabis. The trap is entirely in your mind. The fact that you are your own jailer is an ingenious aspect of the trap and fortunately for you, it's also its fatal flaw.

You have the power to escape simply by understanding the nature of the trap and following the easy instructions in this book.

A CLEVER CON TRICK

When you understand how the cannabis trap works, the solution looks simple: stop taking the drug and just fly away. But as you know, when you're actually in the trap, nothing looks simple. That's because there are two major illusions impairing your judgement:

1. The myth that cannabis gives you pleasure and some kind of benefit
2. The myth that escape will be hard and painful

We'll look at the illusion of pleasure and benefit in more depth later. It's the belief that cannabis gives us some form of pleasure and benefit that makes us think escape will be hard and painful. We fear that stopping will require us to make a sacrifice.

We've all read stories of the suffering and pain that people go through when trying to quit drugs – the repeated visits to rehab, the daily battle to stay clean – it's enough to put you off even trying to quit. And that's all part of the brainwashing.

Quitting IS hard if you go about it the hard way – relying on willpower. Easyway is different. This method makes quitting easy.

It's time we unravelled the illusions that have been keeping you in the cannabis trap.

Chapter 4

SEEING THROUGH THE ILLUSIONS

In most of the Western world, cannabis use is extremely common. The people who come to our live seminars for help come from all walks of life. Cannabis doesn't care whether you're rich or not-so-rich, or just making ends meet. Everyone ends up in the same trap.

You've done an amazing thing. By choosing to read this book, you've ensured your freedom. You've decided you're done with it, it's time to escape from the miserable prison of cannabis addiction, and that's a wondrous thing.

You can stop being so hard on yourself. Don't beat yourself up about your past failed attempts to quit, or what cannabis has done to you and to those you love. It's time to start feeling excited about getting free.

You didn't do anything wrong when you got addicted, you just fell for exactly the same con trick as millions of others. By the end of this book you'll have realised the truth and put all that behind you.

Be clear about this: no-one got free from addiction by focusing on the disadvantages of the drug.

THE BENEFITS OF CANNABIS

Before we can unravel the illusion that cannabis gives us pleasure or some kind of benefit, we need to agree what those benefits are.

Why do we start using cannabis in the first place? To appear more grown up. To be edgy. To appear sophisticated or wild. To rebel. Or to do the opposite – to conform with our peer group. There's a whole host of foolish reasons why we start experimenting with the drug. They probably seem childish and naïve to you now. But don't feel ashamed. Intelligent people fall for confidence tricks. You didn't make a bad investment, or even a bad decision. You were conned.

So you took cannabis and it did seem to live up to the hype.

It seemed to create a sense of inebriation that was different than with booze, deeper or, in the case of stuff like skunk or synths, psychotic.

It appeared to provide some kind of escape, to help you block out life, block out problems, get rid of worries, maybe even ease depression.

It seemed like fun and seemed to help you lose your inhibitions.

You felt high, different, excited.

It seemed to give you confidence and made you feel interesting.

And then it seemed to become a habit.

But the truth is you had already been brainwashed into believing that the drug could do all those things for you.

TV, cinema, rock and roll... everywhere we look we see 'cool' people smoking cannabis or talking about the drug like a walking, talking advertisement for it. From an early age we are primed to expect certain things from the drug. As you now know, all was not as it appeared. In the early days, that is not so easy to see.

We have people tell us the drug seems to affect them in opposite ways. It makes them feel like they are in charge, can get on with their day, be more interesting, talk to anyone about anything. At the same time they say it kills their mind and mood, drains their spirit and energy away and makes them talk a load of nonsense.

The chilled-out rock star image is an amazing mind-trick. The culture of conspicuous drug-taking came out of the shadows of the 1950s and early 1960s and just about the coolest, most "out-there" icons on the planet were the poster boys and girls for the drugs. Bob Dylan, John Lennon, Jimi Hendrix, Mick Jagger, Keith Richards, Janis Joplin, David Bowie, Debbie Harry, Chrissie Hynde... the list goes on. Of course, many of them moved from weed to speed, coke and acid, to heroin, to uppers and downers, all with booze, often all at the same time.

But when you look at these people with open eyes, these superstars of rock and roll, you see reality. Drug-taking didn't make them look cool, or stylish, or sexy, or iconic... THEY made drug-taking look cool, stylish, sexy, and iconic. Take away the drugs and what do you have? Seriously cool, stylish, sexy and iconic superstars.

A procession of those that survived the drug binges now offer sage advice. From Chrissie Hynde (who used Easyway to get free from smoking and alcohol) to Keith Richards, they now openly maintain that dope didn't help them in their creativity or performance, even at the peak of their drug taking. They saw close friends and loved ones have the life sucked out of them, with their spirit and gift and their talent dismantled – the tragedy of addiction.

So much for the pleasure and benefit of cannabis...

THE HIGH

Does cannabis really perk you up? How can it do that and relax you at the same time? It very much depends what you're smoking and what you mix it with, but even if it did act in some kind of stimulating way, phoney stimulants cause huge problems.

You are perfectly well equipped to live your life without the need for false stimulants. Look at youngsters running around at a party with apparently endless energy and excitement. They're on a completely natural energy high, a completely natural emotional high – and that's BEFORE they're plied with chemical- and sugar-laden jelly and ice cream.

As kids we don't need sugar or caffeine or weed to perk us up and have a great time. Put a bunch of youngsters on a soccer pitch with a football and leave them for a few hours and they'll play virtually non-stop. They might pause for a drink from the water fountain but that's it. In most cases they'll play until it's dark. They're on a natural high and their bodies are perfectly equipped to perform at those extraordinary levels. You were like that once. You still are. You just need to treat your body right.

In adulthood too our natural state is to feel energised. As long as you're not sick, you should have more than enough energy to do whatever you want to do in life. If you feel really tired, that's your body asking for sleep and rest, not drugs.

Taking a drug to keep you going is like taking out a payday loan: a quick injection of cash (energy/motivation) and they've got you hooked in, with interest, for the rest of your life, with you having to go back for more and more, again and again, until you do something about it.

Cannabis addiction robs you of your natural energy and makes you permanently tired and exhausted. It probably leads you to overload on caffeine too, which is like pouring petrol on a fire. Take a look at anyone with a caffeine or weed – or a caffeine AND weed – problem; they look tired, run down, lethargic and ready to drop. The irony is, the only thing preventing them from returning to their energetic, athletic, vivacious former self is the very thing they think is helping them; coffee and weed.

We forget how non-dope addicts get through life without having to resort to chemical assistance. They get home from work, it's been a long, hard week and they're committed to going out. They really wanted to go but they're feeling tired and not really up for it. They don't want to let their partner or friends down by cancelling, so they freshen up, maybe take a shower, get changed and emerge for their night out, properly "up for it" and not feeling remotely tired. They're buzzing for the night out now.

Weed addicts can feel that natural energy regeneration too but they credit it to the dope. More often than not, though, a cannabis addict will throw off their work clothes, slump into a chair and smoke the evening away. To hell with their partner who's been dying to go out all week. To hell with the party. To hell with the night out.

Some cannabis users fear that they will have to quit alcohol as well once they are free from dope. That would only be the case if you used the willpower method. When you use willpower to fight an addiction, you're constantly having to resist the temptation to take the drug. After a few drinks that resistance is worn away and you cave in. But with this method you eliminate the temptation, so there is no need or desire to take the drug, no matter how much alcohol you might consume.

A TUG-OF-WAR

There are so many disadvantages to taking dope but you won't get free by focusing on those. Let's face it, you know all about them already: the waste of money, the sleep problems, the fatigue, the lethargy, the lack of drive and vitality.

Addicts know all the downsides but we kid ourselves that there's some sort of pay-off, some amazing benefit to taking the drug that overrides all the downsides. Otherwise why would we keep taking it?

This creates a tug-of-war in our minds between two conflicting fears: on one side the fear of what it's doing to us; on the other side the fear of how miserable life would be without the drug and the benefits it gives us. Whichever aspect we focus on, we feel fear. And it's fear that keeps us hooked. The fears at both ends of that tug of war are caused by one thing: cannabis.

A CRUTCH

I've always had a great analogy for drug addiction of any sort; nicotine, alcohol, cocaine, cannabis, gambling, anything… it's like someone who hasn't got a broken leg buying a crutch that's riddled with woodworm.

The belief that you need cannabis as a crutch is keeping you in the trap.

We had a client – let's call her Beth – who described her life as a dope smoker. If she had a day off she could lose the whole morning as a result of a "wake and bake". She smoked dope every day and felt permanently tired and lethargic, and like many people she relied on coffee to push her through the day.

Beth wasn't wealthy; she was a single mum and her daughter had recently left home to go to college. The financial strain that cannabis was putting on her was immense and she found that it got worse when her daughter went to university. When her daughter lived at home she wouldn't have dreamt of getting high first thing in the morning, but as soon as that control aspect was removed she found herself doing it more and more. She felt she took cannabis to make her feel relaxed and chilled but then would drink gallons of coffee to keep her going. She'd then end up having another joint to calm her down again. In amongst all this she was mixing the cannabis with tobacco: three conflicting chemicals all battling to impact her body and brain.

In truth, all Beth was doing was trying to get back to normal. It was a revelation to her that all she needed to do was stop doing the drugs.

If you think you need dope to help you get through the day, forget it. You'll find your days much more energised and enjoyable once you've got dope out of your life. Tiredness isn't a weakness to be battled with. It's your body telling you that you need to rest. Becoming permanently sluggish because of dope smoking is your body telling you that you're poisoning it, that you need to stop. You override those warning signals at your peril.

Quitting cannabis does not mean giving up partying. In fact, get the thought out of your mind that you're "giving up" anything. On the contrary, you'll be better equipped to party all night, if that's what you want to do.

Beth got in touch soon after her seminar and her message was full of enthusiasm and light. She told us, "I stopped wallowing at home in my sloppy joes, stopped being cocooned in that horrible, demotivating fog and I now enjoy parties more than ever. I've got more energy, I have more fun. Now when I have an evening in on the couch, it's a choice I make to unwind, not a prison cell which I have to return to every night."

Beth's story is just one example of how addiction and drugs are a massive underestimation of our own natural resources and human spirit. As addicts we give the drug way more credit for way more strength than it ever had. The fact is the drug is a cowardly, pathetic confidence trickster, who steals our worth, our strength, our true character and our true selves.

Cannabis gives you no support whatsoever. It makes you think you need support, then takes away your natural ability to support yourself, creating the illusion that you can only get by with the help of the drug.

Apparently there's a tribe somewhere in the world that, if you draw a white chalk circle around one of them, they can't step out of it. They believe so strongly that they must stay in the circle and that belief alone keeps them there. There is absolutely nothing physically holding them in.

You might think that tribe are ignorant, yet you know what it's like to be locked in by a belief. Up until now, you thought it would be hard or even impossible to stop taking cannabis, that life without it would be too miserable to contemplate. Now you need to change your mindset and see that it's fine to step out of the circle.

Nothing bad is going to happen. Quite the reverse, in fact. Only good things lie ahead.

UPS AND DOWNS

Have you noticed how, as you got sucked deeper and deeper into the addiction, the joints got fatter or more frequent? We only feel the need for more of something when what we have is not keeping us satisfied. And that's the case with all drugs. They can never leave you feeling satisfied, because the Little Monster starts grumbling as soon as the drug starts leaving your body. Rather than chasing a high, you're actually trying to constantly shake off a low.

And guess what created that low. Dope! And every joint you have perpetuates rather than relieves it. The sense of relief – the so-called high – is merely an illusion, as I'll explain in the next chapter.

You don't control your cannabis consumption, cannabis controls you. If you had any choice in the matter you wouldn't be reading this book.

We all start taking the drug for a variety of foolish reasons, all of which boil down to the desire to feel good. The fact is there are plenty of things you can do to feel genuinely wonderful. The human brain and body are perfectly capable of finding pleasure and stimulation without resorting to drugs.

As soon as drugs become involved we begin to override our natural ability to feel good, ignore our body's warning signs, push ourselves too far and lose touch with our natural highs. All the really exciting REAL fun soon drains away and we're just left doing the drug day in, day out, never being allowed to stop.

THE WEED WINS.

Even if you only do it once a week, you've still been dragged into the addiction pit. You've become aware, even if it's just at the back of your mind, that you no longer do cannabis because you like it or because you want to, but because something is compelling you, against your better judgement.

Deep down, you know that the "high" you're looking forward to is actually just the relief of a low. It's not genuine fun or pleasure. All you need to do is realise and accept that cannabis created that low and the way to get rid of it is to stop taking cannabis.

The alternative is to stay on the weed and spend the rest of your life trying to shake off that low – which you can never do because you're relying on the one thing that's causing the low. The more you try to shake it off, the more frequent your dope consumption becomes and the further you get from ever feeling the relief you crave.

That is the nature of the trap. It tricks you into seeking relief in the one thing that is dragging you down. We'll explain this further in the next chapter.

Chapter 5

ADDICTION

We need to fix in your mind exactly how the addiction works – how we're fooled into believing that we get some kind of pleasure or benefit from the drug.

The total period of cannabis withdrawal is between about two and five days depending on how much you take, how long you've taken it, your body size and makeup. It can be measured in your system for longer than that but any noticeable withdrawal feelings end after a few days.

A lot of dope addicts go all week, or even several weeks, without taking dope and go through complete withdrawal without even noticing it, the physical withdrawal is so mild. Someone using dope every day just keeps topping it up. Whichever type you are, withdrawal will be easy.

Think of it as that Little Monster that feeds on cannabis and lets out a feeble cry when it doesn't have it. You can destroy the Little Monster simply by starving it to death.

The cries of the Little Monster are so feeble as to be almost imperceptible. It's very easy to ignore them. The problem arises when they arouse the Big Monster.

The Big Monster, which lives in your brain, is the belief that cannabis gives you some sort of genuine pleasure or benefit. As long as you believe that you can't quit without sacrificing something wonderful, the Big Monster will continue to control you.

But killing the Big Monster is easy too. We just need to help you to see cannabis for what it really is, rather than the myth, the illusion, that you've been sold.

It's a combination of that Little Monster (the mild physical addiction) and the Big Monster (the belief that you get something positive from the drug and that it will be hard to stop) that keeps you hooked. Both monsters are at work whether you take the drug every day or twice a month. Deep inside you know you're an addict – otherwise you wouldn't be reading this book. Follow the instructions and you'll see just how easy it is to be free.

THE SLIPPERY SLOPE

We've likened the decline into addiction to the pitcher plant. Actually, the term "slippery slope" is figurative. It's more like a series of ups and downs, where the downs are always greater than the ups. The following text describes it well. It represents the process we go through in becoming addicted and how we're fooled into thinking that we get some kind of boost, or high, from cannabis.

Before you had your first ever joint you were complete. You were not born with a dope deficiency. You were "Normal".

That first ever joint felt like it lifted us above normal, but we need to factor in the lifetime's brainwashing surrounding dope. The excitement, the buzz, the peer pressure, the peer adulation, the rebelliousness of it all. There's no doubt that it makes us feel different, but if you gave that drug, even in its mildest form, to a child who had never had it before and was yet to be brainwashed into believing the hype about it, how do you think it would make them feel? It would be a very unpleasant experience for them.

That first cannabis experience wasn't a high as such. Yes there was a feeling of danger, a feeling of excitement about doing it. And it definitely felt different. Your blood pressure dropped and your heartbeat sped up to compensate for it. Your brain was bombarded by THCs, impairing perception and thought. You bought into the effect.

You were effectively poisoning yourself.

As time passed the physical withdrawal began. If you mixed cannabis with tobacco, you were experiencing withdrawal from two drugs: cannabis and nicotine. The withdrawal for both is identical and mixing them won't make it harder for you to quit. You just need to understand how withdrawal works.

It creates an empty, insecure, unsettled feeling (the Little Monster). You gradually descend below "Normal" for the first time, feeling slightly uncomfortable, slightly unsettled, like something is missing.

Now you have another joint and that slightly empty, insecure, unsettled feeling disappears. You return towards "Normal" again but you don't quite get back there – you've let a serious poison (or two) into your body and it will disrupt and distort the working of your body and brain in a whole variety of ways.

Can you see how the second joint seemed to give you a boost or a high? You did feel better than a moment before but all you did was get rid of the unpleasant feeling caused by the first joint.

As you begin to withdraw from the second joint, the empty, slightly insecure, unsettled feeling returns and you find yourself descending again. A devastating lifetime's chain has started and there are only two things that can end it: stop taking the drug or stop living.

In quite a short space of time, we get used to the empty, insecure, unsatisfied feeling. It starts to feel normal because we spend most of our lives with it – always down below "Normal". Whenever we take the drug, we do feel better than a moment before.

Yet each dose takes us a step further in the addiction, further and further away from normality, further and further away from real pleasure, real highs, real life. Now, on top of the physical withdrawal, you have the mental craving. Because you believe the drug to be a friend, a crutch, a boost and an essential part of being you, you feel miserable without it. But in time you also feel miserable and useless when you've had it.

The longer you go between fixes, the more precious it seems to become. The greater the illusory boost and the more miserable you feel afterwards. The trouble is that this misery, because it creeps up on us over the years, seems normal. How on earth do we consider this deterioration of body, mind and spirit as being normal?

And yet, rather than blame the drug, we blame the circumstances in our lives: the stress of work or home life, our partner, our age, a whole host of things. After a few years in the trap, it's really a triple low that feels like our normal:

1. A very slight physical feeling of withdrawal.
2. The mental craving, causing discontent between doses of the drug.
3. All compounded by the general misery of being an addict and being left helpless in the trap, with all the physical damage that causes to our body and brain.

THE ILLUSION OF PLEASURE

Anything that lifts us from that low, any slight boost, of course it's going to feel like a high, an ally and a crutch. It really isn't any of those things.

The "high" is just a temporary and partial relief from the low that we've come to think of as normal. And don't forget that this is a powerful poison, so its overall effect on your mood, your health and your wellbeing, even if you're a relatively intermittent user, is devastating.

It's time to be honest with yourself. Is the reason you're reading this book testimony to the fact that cannabis has done all sorts of wonderful things for you? Or is it the complete opposite? Isn't it true that, in fact, it's the failure of cannabis to do any of the things it's reputed to do that has brought you to this point?

Start seeing these illusions for what they really are.

The great news is that you get back to "Normal" incredibly quickly. You don't have to wait any time at all. Once you've cut off the supply of the drug to the Little Monster he dies very quickly. The Big Monster dies even faster. It's the Big Monster that keeps you down far below "Normal". But it's dying as you read this book and follow the instructions.

WARNING LIGHTS

Imagine a pilot flying over a mountain range in thick clouds. The plane needs to fly at a certain altitude to avoid the mountains and the pilot gauges the altitude by looking at the altimeter. If the pilot looks at the altimeter and sees that the plane is flying too low, they may feel a momentary surge of panic but they will respond quickly and pull the plane up to a safe height.

The altimeter is the constant gauge of danger from the mountains and as long as it keeps working and the pilot keeps responding, the flight will remain safe.

But suppose the altimeter malfunctions and the little warning light that flashes when the plane drops too low stops working. The pilot thinks everything is fine but really the plane is hurtling towards the mountains with the pilot oblivious to the impending danger.

Some people say that dope helps them to block out their worries, their stress, their concerns. Since when did blocking out problems and worries solve anything? Eventually, when we sober up, the problems haven't gone away. They're still there and, in all likelihood, they've got worse.

"Blocking out" life, worries and problems simply does not work. It deprives us of our natural safety equipment and results in more problems and more worries, not less. When it's an unanticipated consequence of our addiction that's bad enough, but to deliberately take a drug in an attempt to achieve that condition would be the same as the pilot deliberately tampering with the altimeter to ensure that it doesn't work properly.

As a result of reading this book, you won't be losing the ability to block things out, you'll be gaining the ability to see more clearly. And anyway, blocking things out is NOT why you take cannabis. To present it as a reason implies that you have some sort of choice over whether you take the drug or not. If you had any choice you wouldn't be reading this book.

The reason you take the drug is because you're addicted, pure and simple. Any justification you might use for why you take it is simply an excuse – and not one that stands up to scrutiny.

Chapter 6

LAME EXCUSES

As addicts, we try to explain away our inability to quit. We rack our brains to find a reason why, in spite of the obvious disadvantages, we continue to take the drug, against our better judgement. This reinforces the brainwashing about the drug; we conclude, "It must do something for me, otherwise I wouldn't take it." Perversely, the absence of good reasons for taking the drug somehow add to its mystique.

So we concoct lame excuses to mask the real reason why we take cannabis – addiction. Addiction steals the brain's ability to distinguish between real and phoney pleasures, benefits and sensations of relief. It also forces us to lie, to others and to ourselves.

A FALSE FRIEND?

Imagine you met someone new and after you'd got to know them a little they announced that they'd had a bit of luck and come into some money, and they gave you £100. It would be pretty weird – but bear in mind that they insist that they want to share their good fortune and that they really would like you and their other friends to share in their luck. It's £100. It's not going to change your life, but hey, why not go out for a bite to eat or buy something nice for the kids?

Imagine that a month later they did the same. It feels a bit more relaxed this time, you took it last time so why not? You take the £100 and thank them.

Imagine this has happened regularly for a run of months and then, gradually, the £100 seem to be headed your way every few weeks rather than monthly. Then every couple of weeks. Then every week. Every single week this person gives you £100. You would still find it a bit weird, but you would be appreciative and feel indebted to them. You would think of them as an incredibly kind, generous and lovely friend. You would be grateful to them for the help they had given you.

How would you feel if one day you found out that this "friend" had actually been stealing from you. They would take £200 from your bank account and give £100 of it to you. Every single time they had given you £100 they had just taken £200 out of your account without you knowing.

Would you forgive them?

Would you spend time with them any more?

Would you accept any more supposed gifts from them?

Would you feel grateful?

No way! Of course you wouldn't. Not even a little.

So dismiss any feelings of gratitude for anything you think cannabis might have done for you. Whatever 'pleasure' you thought you were getting was fake, phoney, it was deceitful and it made a fool of you. And it stole from you.

But here's a question you may have been pondering over the last chapter. Does it really matter whether the pleasure or benefit you think you get from dope is real or illusory, as long as it feels like a pleasure or benefit?

Would it bother you that you were having your house burgled if you couldn't see it happening? And if the burglar turned out to be someone you thought was a friend? Would that feel ok? Because that's what cannabis is doing to you. Robbing you and laughing at you while you make excuses for it.

Let's look at some of those excuses.

I NEED CANNABIS TO OVERCOME MY SHYNESS

Firstly, what's wrong with shyness? It is not an unattractive trait. Who would you rather spend time with, someone who doesn't talk much but listens, or someone who talks too much and shows no interest in what you have to say? OK, social occasions may make shy people feel vulnerable but taking dope to numb that feeling is like the pilot tampering with the altimeter. You increase your chances of crashing and burning socially. On dope you're much more vulnerable to being seen as boring, repetitive and inane, and making those around you wish you'd go away. What's appealing about that?

Cannabis doesn't make us have more fun or make us more interesting, it just removes our ability to tell when we're being dull, oafish and obnoxious. In fact, many of the people reading this book will have that as one of their primary reasons for wanting to get free.

CANNABIS DOESN'T GIVE YOU ANY SOCIAL POWERS OR ADVANTAGES OR BENEFITS – IT TAKES ALL YOUR POWERS AWAY.

You don't take dope because it helps you lose your inhibitions, you take IT IN SPITE OF THAT. You don't take dope because it helps you have fun, you've forgotten how to have fun BECAUSE you take dope.

That's why you're reading this book.

GETTING HIGH IS FUN

When we first start doing cannabis it feels like the greatest adventure imaginable. The rebelliousness of it, the decadence of it, the thrill of the moment that first time – very few people take it in their stride. No wonder we think it felt amazing.

And in truth there was something there: a change in your brain and body; but the expectation of it being amazing almost guaranteed it would feel that way. Give cannabis to a youngster who has no knowledge of the drug and they would describe a deeply unpleasant and uncomfortable experience.

Of course you'll remember occasions when you had fun when you've been high – especially if it's one of the occasions you didn't ruin because you were high. But whatever occasions spring to mind, those occasions are equally fun, equally thrilling, equally amazing without the drug. In fact, they are more so. Rediscovering true sensations, true connections to loved ones, true pleasure, is exquisite.

Perhaps you have doubts about that.

If so, remember how much fun children have without any chemical assistance? Then look at the amazing, wonderful, magical aspects of life that have nothing to do with dope: love, sex, dancing, exploring the countryside, or a city, sport, reading, movies, theatre, dining out, catching up with old friends, music or just the mindful appreciation and enjoyment of the beauty of the world around you... and so many pleasures.

Then think about any occasion where lots of people are having fun. It could be a huge sporting event, a huge musical event, a huge wedding or a big party, they all have one thing in common: most of the people there, having fun, letting their hair down, letting themselves go, letting themselves feel amazing and wonderful and excited, are not using dope.

It's time to put behind you the idea that dope is your doorway to fun. In fact, dope keeps that doorway shut. To open it again, you need to reconnect you to the real you, not the dope-addicted, used-up, messed-up version of you.

DOPE GIVES ME CONFIDENCE

You may think that overcoming shyness and attaining self-confidence are the same thing, but there are differences. In both cases, however, using dope to change your mindset is like the low-flying pilot tampering with the gauges.

It's certainly not an argument for doing the drug. In fact, it's quite the reverse. People who use dope to build their confidence usually end up making fools of themselves at best or sustaining serious harm at worst. It's not confidence you're building, it's OVER-confidence. And can you think of a single significant moment in your life, or anyone else's, when it might be an advantage to be over-confident?

There aren't any.

Ask any sports coach; over-confidence is a terrible, debilitating, destructive thing. It has led to the loss of epic sporting battles, as well as actual battles and careers. Confidence is the stuff of champions and winners; over-confidence is the stuff of losers, braggarts and fools. And it's a thin line between the two, which requires a keen self-awareness – not a strong point for anyone doped off their head.

Inhibitions are healthy. They keep us safe and allow us to act in the best interests of our wellbeing. At the top of a tall building, it's a feeling of inhibition, of insecurity, that protects us from going too close to the edge and endangering ourselves.

When we interfere with our natural instincts we cause ourselves tremendous problems. Instead of feeling a little insecure in a secure situation, we have a joint and feel overly secure in what has now become an insecure situation.

Whether it's a situation where you're in mortal danger at the top of a tall building or whether you feel overconfident before making a speech and forget your lines as soon as you stand up, the pitfalls are serious. The fact that the drug makes you "feel" confident only takes away your awareness of your limitations in any given situation, and that is a recipe for disaster.

I CAN TAKE IT OR LEAVE IT

First of all, that's a strange reason for doing anything you claim to enjoy. If you asked a singer why she sings, you'd be taken aback if she said, "I can take it or leave it." It's hardly a positive reason, is it?

Neither is it a valid one. It's important to quash the belief that you could be someone who can take or leave the drug.

You may have friends who seem to be able to dabble with cannabis here and there, just having a couple of joints every now and then. These dabblers come in various types. Firstly, there are the ones who just lie. They'll tell you that they only have the occasional puff but they always seem to be puffing away whenever you see them. They lie to you and they lie to themselves.

Then there are the rank amateurs, who smoke it maybe a few times a year. They don't really get much out of it, they just do it for the show. They run the risk of becoming a full-on dope addict yet claim they chose to take it or leave it.

Don't envy them. You were like that once. Now you know what dope addiction can do to you, can you think of anything more stupid than someone who remains in the state whereby they can take or leave it, when they could just leave it?

Then there are dope addicts who either can't afford to take more or they're so terrified of what it would do to them that they force themselves not to take it every day. They are fighting, day in, day out, using tremendous willpower to limit their intake of the drug. It's a miserable existence; they're miserable when they can't do it and miserable when they can.

Don't envy them. It's like being on a permanent diet.

Their "take it or leave it" level of dope taking, which may look to you like control, only works while the restraint lasts. Sooner or later, though, it disintegrates.

Dabblers battle to limit their intake for a variety of reasons. They might be terrified of the effect on their work, mind, body and/or relationships. Take those concerns out of the equation and they go berserk. They're the people who go nuts on holiday or at parties, where any checks on their behaviour are removed.

They're all suffering and if you recognise yourself in any of the characters described, please don't worry. Freedom is in your grasp and you don't need to feel anxious about any of this stuff anymore. Just remember:

NEVER ENVY OTHER DOPE ADDICTS.

IT'S JUST A HABIT I'VE GOT INTO

That's another strange argument.

"You play golf?"

"Yeah, I play golf."

"You enjoy it?"

"Well, it's just a habit really."

If it's just a habit and you know it's causing you misery, why not break the habit?

The fact is, despite the frequent use of the word habit when referring to addiction, you don't take cannabis out of habit. There may be habits that are associated with your dope taking, but the reason you keep taking dope is because you're addicted and it's essential that you understand the difference. Otherwise you won't fully grasp the nature of the trap and you will remain vulnerable.

Certain repeated behaviours become habitual, often for reasons of convenience, efficiency or conformity. In the UK, we always drive on the left. We don't have to think about it, we're in the habit of pulling out onto the left-hand side of the road. If we travel to Europe, where they drive on the right we adjust with ease. And when we return home, we readjust just as easily. Habits are easy to break as long as you want to break them. With habits you are in control.

Addiction is confused with habit because it involves the same repetitive actions and there is a level of unconsciousness about it, i.e. we don't stop to think about what we're doing. But the force that compels you to smoke dope is not a logical reasoning, as it is with driving on the same side of the road or sitting in the same seat on the train to work every day, it's a feeling of physical unease from withdrawal coupled with a mental belief that dope is the only thing that can relieve it.

That's how addiction works: it deludes you into seeking relief by taking more of the thing that's causing you misery.

We get into habits because they provide us with a genuine benefit. With addiction, we think there's a benefit but it's illusory. When we take our heads out of the sand and list all the advantages and disadvantages of taking cannabis, there is only one conclusion:

"I'm a mug; it's time to stop!"

And that's why, as addicts, we feel instinctively stupid deep down inside.

But addicts are not stupid. They've been fooled by a powerful force called addiction.

After you've finished this book, the habits that you associate with your dope taking might lead the thought to flash into your mind, "I'll have a joint now". It might appear to be an important part of your ritual when you come home from work, or during your preparations for a day out or a night on the town. Because your dope addiction has required you to use dope at those times it appears to have become part of those rituals, and when you quit those other habits might have you think of taking dope. If so, there is no need to be alarmed.

In the past, when you tried to use willpower to quit, such a thought would have opened up the floodgates of desperation and desire and led to a battle that you were destined to lose. But with Easyway, the need and desire for the drug are eliminated, making those moments easy to brush aside. In fact, they become moments of real pleasure as you remind yourself how lucky you are to be free.

So be clear about this: the habit of taking dope didn't get you addicted; being addicted to dope got you into the habit of taking it. Please read that sentence again – it's important that you see your descent into addiction accurately. You'd be amazed how many people mistakenly believe they got into the habit of using dope and it is that which addicted them.

Escape the addiction and any habitual issues and triggers are easy and enjoyable to deal with.

Chapter 7

WILLPOWER

Just as the willpower method is commonly assumed to be the only way to cure an addiction, those who fail to quit that way and remain in the trap are generally branded as weak willed. Indeed, they brand themselves as such. They assume it is they who have failed, not the method.

If that's why you feel you've failed to quit up until now – because you lack the strength of will – then you haven't yet understood the nature of the trap you're in. Ask yourself if you're weak willed in other areas of your life. Perhaps you eat too much or you drink too much and consider this to be further evidence that you lack willpower.

There is a connection between all addictions but the connection is not that they are signs of lack of willpower. On the contrary, they're more likely signs of a strong will. What they all share is that they are traps created by misleading information and untruths. And one of the most misleading untruths of all is that quitting requires willpower.

HOW WEAK-WILLED ARE YOU?

There are probably plenty of examples in your life of how you possess huge amounts of willpower. In fact, it's normally strong-willed people who end up addicted to drugs. It takes a strong willed person to persist in doing something that goes against all their instincts and turn a blind eye to all the potential downsides of the addiction.

And think of the lengths you go to in order to get hold of dope. When you want it, you want it, and you'd go to extraordinary lengths to obtain it.

When you persist in doing something even though it's clearly not in your best interests, that's not weak willed, it's wilful. If you tried to open a door by pushing on the hinge side and someone pointed out that you'd find it easier if you pushed on the handle side, you would have to be pretty stubborn to ignore them. A weak-willed person would take the path of least resistance.

With the willpower method you force yourself into a self-imposed tantrum, like a child being deprived of its toys. When that happens, the child experiences the most violent physical symptoms, in the same way that most addicts do when they attempt to quit using willpower. It might have surprised you to learn that the physical withdrawal from cannabis is actually very mild and doesn't require a great struggle to overcome. It's what goes on in your mind that causes the physical discomfort.

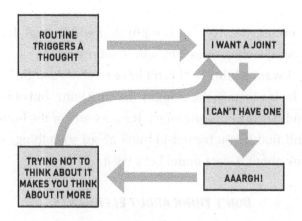

REWIRING YOUR BRAIN

This diagram helps to explain what might have happened in the past when you tried to quit dope using willpower. And hopefully it will explain how easy it is for you to change your mindset, essentially rebooting, resetting your mind back to pre-addiction mode.

In the past when you tried to quit cannabis your experience went a little like this: You get home from work or go to a friend's house or a party or somewhere that previously you would have had a joint. Suddenly the thought pops into your mind, "I want a joint". You fight it back, trying to put the thought out of your mind. But the next thought you have is "I can't have one" which carries the physical response, "Aaargh!" It's a gut-wrenching feeling – although, to keep it in perspective, it's not torture. Neither is it physical withdrawal. It is a physical feeling caused by a thought process.

"I want a joint" » "I can't have one"» "Aaargh!"

Trying to push the thought "I want a joint" out of your mind has the opposite effect. It's a feature of the human mind that if you try not to think about something, you think about it even more! Let's try it.

DON'T THINK ABOUT ELEPHANTS.

What's the first thing that popped into your mind?

So the thought of taking dope stays on your mind and it triggers the thought again, "I want a joint", then the next thought, "I can't", followed by that horrible "Aaargh!" feeling again. On each cycle the "Aaargh!" feeling gets worse and worse, as you try not to think about it but think about it even more!

"I want a joint" » "I can't" » "Aaargh!" No wonder you've found it hard to break free in the past. It's almost guaranteed to fail.

UNDERSTAND YOUR THOUGHTS

By the time you finish this book you'll understand that there are no benefits, advantages or pleasures to be gained from taking dope. Once you've established that, the only natural thought for you to have when you think about the drug is, "Great – I'm FREE!"

You'll feel no sense of deprivation because you'll understand that there is no point in taking cannabis. Nothing to be gained at all. And this time, when you get home from work, or round your friend's house, or to the party, or wherever you might have had a joint before, the habitual thought "I want a joint" might pop into your head, but your reaction won't be "I can't", it will be:

"GREAT – I'M FREE!"

You won't have to try "not to think about" cannabis, because the more you think about it, the more you're reminded of your freedom, the happier you'll be.

So for a little while after quitting you just need to give yourself the space to acknowledge what's going on in your mind. If one of those habitual thoughts pops into your head and you catch yourself thinking "I want a joint", or even "I can't", rather than worrying about it or battling to force it out of your mind, embrace the moment and use it as a reminder of what you've escaped from. Take pleasure in the knowledge that you no longer have to respond to those habitual thoughts by taking cannabis. You are free.

Right now, you might find it hard to believe that you will ever feel that way, but remember, the horrible, angsty "Aaargh!" feeling you've experienced in the past has nothing to do with withdrawal, it's all about what's going on in your head. Removing the brainwashing feels incredible and turns moments of potential misery into moments of pure joy.

As you read this book you're getting rid of the "want" so there is no genuine "I want a joint", only habitual thoughts that are easy to process. You will no longer regard yourself as weak-willed.

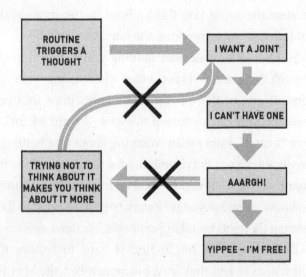

Remember, strong-willed high achievers fall into the addiction trap: business executives, sports stars, politicians. You don't take dope because you're weak willed, you take dope because you're addicted to it. The great news is that the addiction is easy to break.

All you need to do is follow the instructions.

THE TUG-OF-WAR OF FEAR

A feature common to all addictions is the tug of war going on in the addict's mind. On one side is all the known harm caused by the addiction: the health scares, it costs a fortune, it enslaves us, it corrupts our emotions, it drives away friends and family, it leaves us feeling lousy, it damages the brain. On the other side of the tug of war is the fear that we couldn't cope without the drug. How could we enjoy life, handle social occasions, handle work and stress, carry on with our lives?

More simply, it's the fear of what will happen to us if we carry on taking dope versus the fear of what will happen if we stop. Two very real fears on either end of the rope. Both caused by cannabis addiction! Do you recognise that conflict? It never occurs to us as addicts that the fears at both ends of the tug-of-war are caused by the same thing: dope. We seek comfort in cannabis because of the way addiction works but we're mistaken.

DOPE DOESN'T RELIEVE THE FEAR, IT CAUSES IT.

Imagine if you could get rid of both fears. The dope would lose its grip. Forever. So let's look at those fears.

The fear caused by your knowledge of the harm that dope is doing to you will be removed the moment you stop taking it. That's great news. The fear of what life will be like without dope – after you've quit – will disappear as you continue to read this book.

The scare stories you've heard about how hard it is to quit and the bad experiences you've had in the past when you tried to quit on our own are all based on one thing: the willpower method. The people you've seen struggle and fail to get free – you included – were trying to do it the hard way. This way is different. Hopefully you're sensing that already. If not, don't worry – you will.

The belief that life is more fun, or more chilled, on dope is a myth, which we have already disproven. There is nothing to fear from life without dope. Only marvellous gains and an incredible feeling of:

FREEDOM!

If you still find that hard to imagine, no problem. All you need to do is carry on reading and follow all the instructions.

Chapter 8

COME TO YOUR SENSES

We've examined some of the misconceptions around what cannabis does for you. Now let's shift the emphasis a little and ask, "What's so great about being a stoner?"

Apart from providing momentary relief from withdrawal, doesn't it simply deprive you of the ordinary use of your senses and reason? In fact, dope affects all our faculties, including self-control.

Most people have a checkpoint between brain and mouth that keeps them out of trouble. Dope short-circuits this, even more so when combined with alcohol or other drugs. It reduces inhibition, and that is not useful, positive or desirable. It makes us behave in all sorts of ways that we wouldn't dream of if we were thinking straight.

You might protest that you're a perfectly civilised human being when you're stoned but it's likely that one of the reasons you're reading this book is because you know deep down that you're not. There's plenty about your addiction that makes you feel bad.

THE SOCIAL LUBRICANT

If you feel that dope helps you enjoy social situations, maybe you feel the real you is a little restrained or shy. You can overcome that reservation by making a habit of helping other people overcome theirs. Most people love talking about themselves. So ask them questions – about their job, their interests, their kids. They'll think you're a great conversationalist when you've hardly said a word! And there's no gut-wrenching regret about your behaviour the next morning.

If you're so shy that this suggestion fills you with panic, take comfort in this: shyness can be a very attractive quality. People would much rather spend time with someone who is a bit shy than listen to the hollow boasts of some sweaty, high pot-head, who makes no sense.

Are we ever fooled by a stoner? Do we regard them as dynamic, courageous types, facing up to life's big challenges? Or do we see them as a little bit sad, a little bit inadequate, forever leaning on that woodworm-riddled crutch?

The sad thing is that everyone knows it's just an act, with the possible exception of the person under the influence at the time. While you're stoned you feel invincible and like you rule the world. The trouble with using drugs in this way is that you're telling yourself your inner resources don't exist. If, for example, you resort to that kind of 'courage', you're telling yourself that you lack real courage. After a while you start to believe it and act as if it were true.

Do you really want that phoney sense of 'confidence'? Or is it the fact that you're sick of it that has brought you to this point? The fact is, you probably know how weird and phoney and tired and used up you feel when you're doped up.

And it scares the life out of you.

THE ROLE OF COURAGE

Genuine courage is not feeling no fear, it's taking the decision to act in spite of fear.

The proverbial ostrich buries its head in the sand at the first sign of danger. It's removing fear but it's not removing the danger. In fact, it's making itself more vulnerable to the danger.

Cannabis can, in certain situations, temporarily reduce fear but only by diminishing your instinct for danger, not by giving you courage. Therefore, resorting to dope in such a situation would actually prevent you from summoning the full force of your own inner courage.

Courage is like a muscle: the more you use it, the bigger it grows and the easier it becomes to use. The ostrich becomes more vulnerable because it deprives itself of three other faculties essential for survival: the ability to see, to fight and to run.

Cannabis has a similar effect. It impairs your vision and judgement, confuses your instinct to fight or flee and impairs physical coordination.

A firefighter who runs into a burning building doesn't need weed to give them courage. In fact, weed would render them less effective and more vulnerable. Remember the pilot flying over a mountain range in fog? If you've ever had to drive in fog you'll know it's an alarming experience, even at the slowest speed in daylight. Imagine what it must be like to fly a plane through a mountain range in night time fog. Now try and imagine what it would be like if the pilot suddenly realised the radar, altimeter, fuel gauge and compass were malfunctioning. How terrifying would that be?

But can you imagine the pilot deliberately tampering with those instruments, so they give false readings? The plane is flying through fog in a range where the peaks reach four thousand feet. The altimeter registers the plane's altitude at two thousand feet: so the pilot adjusts its calibration so that it reads five thousand feet. That's effectively what we're doing when we smoke dope to mask our fear.

If you knew the situation required you to employ your mental and/or physical faculties, the fear would be increased. Why? Because while an ostrich might fool itself by burying its head in the sand, the pilot would know that by interfering with the instrument panel they have placed themselves in even greater danger. So in this case the fear would be magnified. The only way the pilot could remove the fear would be to take action: to increase the altitude.

In fairness to ostriches, it's a myth that they bury their heads in times of danger. Any species that adopted such a stupid tactic would be highly unlikely to survive.

THE SENSE OF FEAR

Like all animals, we are completely dependent on our senses and instincts. We think of fear, inhibition, stress and nerves as debilitating evils, but they are vital components of our instinctive survival mechanism. Use a drug to meddle with them and you're embarking on a course as suicidal as the pilot who tinkers with the altimeter.

There are people born without normal instincts: without inhibition and fear, without any qualms about harming themselves or others. They act like the worst kind of drug addict, even when they're sober. Most of them are in institutions, for their own good and that of society.

There are also people born without senses: completely blind and deaf, with no sense of taste, touch or smell.

Would you envy such a person? Would you get in a car with a blind driver at the wheel?

People who live with disabilities are aware of their limitations and adjust accordingly, whereas even small amounts of cannabis will impair your faculties infinitely more than you realise at the time.

Fear is the instinct that stops us in our tracks, makes us think twice, self-evaluate, moderate our behaviour. Without fear, we put ourselves in danger, whether that's genuine physical danger or the threat of social exclusion. The problem with drugs like dope is that they fool us into thinking we're being cool when the opposite is actually true. They inhibit the senses that enable us to adjust our behaviour, to gauge the mood, to apply tact, to grasp opportunities for a witty remark, to charm.

Sometimes we're like the ostrich, kidding ourselves there is no danger when there patently is; in others, we're like the pilot who has tampered with the instruments. In some situations dope takes away anxiety when we need it, in others it increases anxiety when there is no need. On dope we become fearful for no good reason. We call it paranoia.

Imagine you're in the middle of a joint when you receive a call from your boss or an important client or a relative. They have a serious problem and are looking to you for help. At that point you become the pilot: your anxiety would be increased because you would know that you are not in a fit state to solve the problem. You would also have to go through that embarrassing farce of pretending to be in control, when it is blatantly obvious that you're not.

Think of your acquaintances. Who are some of the most stressed and nervous? Aren't they the people who use drugs such as cannabis, cocaine, alcohol and nicotine to try and cope with stress and nerves? Not only do the drugs not help achieve that, they actually make the situations worse.

But a little bit of stress and nerves can be useful as a stimulus to take action. They're part of the human security system. We treat nerves as if they're a disease, rather than a healthy faculty of a fully functional human being. If the door slams and we jump, we tend to say, "Oh! My nerves are bad!" But that's actually a sign of good nerves.

Have you noticed how nervy birds are when feeding? The slightest sound sends them to the safety of the trees. That sound might be a cat. It's not only natural for birds to react like that, it's essential to their survival.

And stress is no more evil than a fire alarm. If something's got you worried, that's an early warning signal and a cue to act. It was your anxiety about your dope addiction that made you turn to this book in the first place. And this is the most important point of all:

IF DOPE WAS MAKING YOU CONFIDENT
AND BRAVE, DO YOU THINK YOU'D
STILL BE READING THIS?

Dope and alcohol may take the edge off inhibitions, fear, nerves and stress in the moment but it magnifies them many times over the morning after. That's not to say dope is always responsible for the actual situation that's causing anxiety (although that is often the case), but it's dope that makes the situation seem like a big deal, rather than a challenge you take in your stride.

I WISH I COULD JUST CUT DOWN

Because we assume there are such things as 'normal' dope users – and that, at one point, we perhaps felt we were one – we think that if we can get back into the "habit" of just having a couple of joints every now and then we'll be able to keep it at that level. People cling to that theory for years, as week-in week-out they prove it to be an impossible myth.

Every addict tries cutting down at some point. You've probably tried before. Did it work? Did it make you a happy dope user, fully in control of your intake?

Or did it make you feel even more addicted than ever? Cutting down doesn't work because that's not how drug addiction works. You don't become less addicted. As long as you keep feeding it, it makes you want to take more and more.

So what would be your ideal intake? One joint a week? Why not three or four? What the question really amounts to is which joint is the point of no return beyond which it's hard not to have another and another and another? Is it the third? If so, why not the fourth or second? And surely it depends on the fatness of the joint. Besides, how can you gauge that point when your judgement has been affected by a drug?

But let's assume you could and you work out that this particular joint, of this particular strength is the one that does the damage. So your rule tonight is two skinny spliffs and no more. The trouble is those two spliffs would make you care a hell of a lot less about the consequences of dope. So what's to stop you saying, "Stuff the rules! I'm having another"?

Anyone who's tried to cut down will know it never lasts, because cannabis consumption is not a habit, it's drug addiction. You become increasingly tolerant to the drug and need more and more to achieve the same effect. Even to maintain your current level you'd have to use willpower for the rest of your life. But let's imagine for a moment that you were capable of doing that. Let's imagine you could use self-discipline and limit yourself to say one joint per week. Wouldn't your whole life become dominated by that one joint?

Why would you want to put yourself through the agony of that? Do you really want to spend the rest of your life wishing it away for your next fix?

Think about it: does dieting make food seem less precious, or a thousand times more so? And how long do you think the average diet lasts? Weeks? Days? Hours? Minutes?

So if it can be that difficult to control your intake of food, which *doesn't* mess with your mind (let's not get onto sugar addiction at this point), how could you possibly hope to control the intake of a drug that removes self-control, self-awareness, caution and care? It's futile to attempt to exercise control over your dope consumption.

More importantly, once you know the truth about the addiction, it's entirely undesirable to attempt to do so.

Everyone who reads this book does so for one of two reasons: either they've proved to themselves that they can't cut down or control their cannabis consumption; or they're just about holding on to being able to do so, albeit with the odd blip, but it's such hell they can't take it anymore. In either case, it's probably dawned on them that they'd rather be completely free. Cutting down is not an option. But that's not a problem, because there are no advantages to consuming *any* amount of cannabis, so you have absolutely nothing to lose by stopping completely.

DOPE MAKES MY PROBLEMS GO AWAY

Does it really? Is dope really a magic balm that makes everything all right? When some charmless stoner is being obnoxious at a party, what do you think? Quick, give him some more dope? Would that lighten him up? Of course not.

The trouble with addictive drugs is that they get even less 'effective' as you develop tolerance, just as rats develop a tolerance to rat poison. Tolerance is the process of the mind and body getting used to dope. You become increasingly resistant to the effect of the drug, so to feel that same effect you need to take more and more, as it becomes less and less effective. That's the way addiction works.

You don't need to list all the problems that have been caused by you taking dope, but can you think of a single problem that was solved by it?

OK, you can no doubt think of occasions that you've really enjoyed while you were on dope, but were they enjoyable because of the dope? Or was it because you were in good company, or there was great music, or entertainment, or the setting was spectacular or the weather was perfect? Do you ever look back and reminisce about evenings that were unforgettable because of the sheer quality of the dope?

Booze and dope are prevalent in our society. For many people, a social event without alcohol sounds like a contradiction in terms and for some the same applies without dope. But if a group of friends are enjoying themselves at a birthday or wedding celebration, it's not because they're consuming alcohol and/or dope. It's because they're having a great time with people whose company they enjoy.

There's a similar atmosphere of joviality and fun in the changing room before a football match, without any alcohol or dope having been consumed. And after the match, does the winning team need alcohol or dope to be happy? No, they're on a genuine high from the moment the game ends. Often they don't even drink the Champagne that's passed around – they squirt it over each other instead!

By the same token, does the atmosphere in the losers' changing room switch from gloom to delight when they have a drink and a doobie? No, the disappointment lingers.

Paul Merson and Tony Adams, two of the leading English football players of the 1980s and 1990s, nearly lost their lives to the motto: "Win or lose, on the booze!" For Paul that normally included drugs too. Paul and Tony were two giants of sport, two supremely skilled, highly competitive, high-achieving, international athletes who were not just compromised by booze and drugs but were bought to their knees, leaving them bawling their eyes out in public, leaving them alone, penniless and lost. There is nothing glamorous about addiction. It steals everything.

The fact that both men have survived and rebuilt their lives, is testimony to their spirit and to the support that surrounds them.

WILL I HAVE TO QUIT ALCOHOL TOO?

We've talked a lot about the link between dope and alcohol and perhaps you're worried that you might have to avoid alcohol after you've quit cannabis. That is not at all necessary. It's a personal decision. You can carry on doing exactly what you normally do, minus the cannabis.

The really important thing is that you don't substitute. In other words, don't drink more than usual in an attempt to replace cannabis.

The caveat to this is if you feel you have a

serious drinking issue that you also want to resolve. If that is the case and you feel confident and empowered after reading this book, by all means commit to leaving alcohol behind as well. If, at some point in the future, you feel that alcohol is causing you concern, we can help you with that too.

NOTHING TO GIVE UP

When you have a great time, don't give the credit to cannabis. Look at the elements that made that occasion so enjoyable. The company, the food, the chat, the laughter, sense of belonging, the entertainment, the location... Ask yourself whether it would have been enjoyable if you'd taken those elements away and just left the dope. In fact many people will be reading this book because weed has robbed them of all those precious elements and left them trapped in a one-dimensional world: sitting around at home... stoned.

It's important to be able to distinguish genuine pleasures from the false pleasure we think we get from dope. The fabulous news is that after you've finished reading this book you'll be free of cannabis and that will allow you to enjoy more good times. You don't have to stop partying and having fun. You're not giving up living. In fact, you're not giving up anything at all. What you are actually doing is getting rid of a disease: cannabis addiction.

Imagine what the effects of cannabis would be like to someone who had never heard of it; somebody who had never been brainwashed or warned about the way the drug changes the way they feel and had never had the chance to build up a tolerance to them. Imagine they were tricked into consuming a large amount of dope and suddenly found themselves unable to think, move, see or talk properly!

Do you think they would enjoy the experience and think all their problems had been taken away?

Of course not.

Chapter 9

THE INCREDIBLE MACHINE

Imagine being a passenger on that flight through fog over mountains and noticing that the pilot is smoking a big fat spliff. Would that reassure you or scare the living daylights out of you?

Think of your body as the plane and you're the pilot. The human body is a highly complex machine, a finely balanced mixture of hormones that regulate our behaviour for our own survival. Your brain is an incredibly sophisticated computer that controls it all, more powerful and complex than anything you'll find in the most modern aeroplane.

Do you really believe you can improve on something that ingenious by taking a chemical that radically affects its proper functioning? If it unnerves you to think of a pilot picking his way through mountains while doped up, why is it OK to do it to yourself?

We're given incredibly strong bodies. Unfortunately we tend to mistreat them terribly. We poison them with drugs, avoid exercise, we overwork, deprive ourselves of sleep, eat junk and gain weight, whilst simultaneously starving ourselves of real nutrition. Some people do all these things and more for years. For decades.

Yet our bodies keep going, in spite of the abuse we subject them to. What an incredible piece of machinery the human body is! And how much more incredible it can be when we treat it with respect.

When we're young adults we're aware of the physical power and strength of our bodies but as we grow a little older we become physically and mentally weaker. We know that our lifestyle is probably not helping; that we could eat more healthily, get more sleep and rest, avoid drinking too much, avoid drugs.

But we've been brainwashed into accepting some kind of decline into old age, in some cases when we're not even out of our 20s or 30s. Just pause for a moment to consider the incredible strength, power and sophistication of our bodies. Think about the thousands of tasks that our bodies perform automatically, all at the same time, even as we sleep.

The heart has to keep pumping, never missing a single beat. Blood must carry oxygen, energy and nutrients to every part of the body. Our internal thermostat has to maintain our body temperature at the correct level. Every one of our organs, including the liver, lungs and kidneys, have to continue to function in harmony. The stomach must digest our food. The intestines must distinguish between food and waste, extract the former and arrange disposal of the latter.

Any good doctor will tell you that your greatest ally in fighting infection and disease is not the doctor or any drugs they can prescribe, but your immune system, which, while all the above functions are being carried out, automatically supplies chemicals such as adrenalin and dopamine to whatever part of your body needs them, in the exact quantities required.

Our knowledge of the human body has expanded a thousandfold in the last one hundred years. We can transplant organs and achieve mind-boggling results with genetic engineering. However, the greatest experts on these subjects admit that this increased insight into the functioning of the human body makes them realise how little we understand about the workings of that incredible machine.

EQUIPPED TO SURVIVE

If your highly sophisticated computer developed a fault, would you let a gorilla try to fix it? All too often it has been shown that, in the long run, the interventions that we undertake with our limited knowledge cause many more problems than they solve.

The human body is by far the most powerful survival machine on the planet. It's a million times more sophisticated than the most powerful spacecraft made by mankind. If we abused our cars as we abused our bodies over the years, they would break down and need to be scrapped in no time at all.

The human body is the culmination of over three billion years of trial and error, all designed to achieve one object and one object alone:

SURVIVAL.

Three billion years is an awful lot of research and when so-called intelligent man contradicts the laws of nature, without knowing the exact consequences of his actions, he is certainly not being intelligent.

Our every instinct and guiding force is to ensure that we survive. It's that instinct that has had you question your consumption of cannabis.

We think of tiredness and pain as evils. In reality, they're essential red warning lights. Tiredness is your body telling you that you need to rest. Pain is telling you that part of your body is being attacked and that remedial action is necessary.

We think of hunger and thirst as evils. In reality, they're essential alarm bells: your body warning you that unless you eat and drink, you will not survive. Each of our senses is designed to ensure that we survive. We're equipped with eyes to see danger, ears to hear danger, a nose to smell it, touch to feel hot or sharp surfaces and taste to know the difference between food and poison.

Many doctors have now discovered that drugs like Valium, Xanax, other Benzodiazepines and medication cause more problems than they solve. These drugs have a similar effect to alcohol. They might take the person's mind off their problems but they don't cure them. When the effect of the drug has worn off, another dose is required. Because the drugs themselves are addictive poisons, they have physical and mental side effects and the body builds an immunity to the drug so that its blocking effect is reduced.

The addict now has the original stress, anxiety and other issues plus the additional physical and mental stress caused by feeling dependent on the drug that is supposed to be relieving the stress and anxiety.

Eventually the body builds such an immunity to the drug that it ceases even to give the illusion of relieving stress. All too often the remedy is now either to administer larger and more frequent doses of the drug, or to subject the patient to an even more potent and dangerous drug. The whole process is an ever-accelerating plunge down a bottomless pit.

Some doctors still defend such drugs by maintaining that they prevent the patient from having a nervous breakdown in the short term. Again they focus on removing the symptoms.

A nervous breakdown isn't a disease. On the contrary, it's a partial cure and another red warning light. It's nature's way of saying, "I can't cope with any more stress, responsibility or problems. I've had it up to here. I need a rest. I need a break."

The problem is that many people often take on too much responsibility. Everything is fine whilst they're in control and can handle it. In fact, they often thrive on it. But everyone has phases in their life when a series of problems coincide. Observe politicians when they're campaigning to become President or Prime Minister. They are strong, rational, decisive and positive. They have simple solutions to all of our problems. But when they achieve their ambition, you can hardly recognise them as the same person. Now that they have the actual responsibility of office, they become negative and hesitant.

No matter how weak or strong we are, we all have bad patches in our lives. The usual tendency at such times is to seek solace through what we've been brainwashed to regard as our traditional crutches: alcohol, nicotine, cannabis and other drugs. It may be usual but there's absolutely nothing rational about it. The only answer to stress is to remove the cause. It's pointless trying to pretend that stress doesn't exist. Whether it is real or illusory, drugs will only make the reality and the illusion worse.

HANDLING STRESS

Another problem is that we are brainwashed into believing that we lead very stressful lives. The truth is that the human species has already successfully removed most of the causes of genuine stress. We no longer have the fear of being attacked by wild animals every time we leave our homes and the vast majority of us don't have to worry about where our next meal will come from or whether we'll have a roof over our heads.

Imagine being a rabbit. Every time you pop your head out of the burrow, you not only have the problem of searching for food for yourself and your family, but you have to avoid becoming the next meal of another creature. Even back in your burrow you can't relax or feel secure, as you're at risk from floods, ferrets and a myriad of other hazards – not to mention those imposed by mankind.

The stress of serving in the Vietnam War understandably caused many servicemen to turn to drugs. But they served for a comparatively short period. How does a rabbit survive Vietnam levels of stress its entire life, yet still manage to procreate at a prolific rate and feed its family? The average rabbit even looks considerably happier than the average human being!

The reason that rabbits can take all this stress and trauma in their stride is because they have adrenalin and other drugs occurring naturally. They also benefit from possessing the powers of sight, smell, hearing, touch, taste and instinct – everything they need to survive. Rabbits are extraordinary survival machines:

BUT THEY'RE NOT AS EXTRAORDINARY AS HUMAN BEINGS.

We have reached a stage of evolution whereby we can even partly control the elements. Properly organised, we could virtually eliminate the effects of droughts, floods and earthquakes. We really have just one substantial enemy to conquer:

OURSELVES.

At our stop smoking seminars we ask smokers, "Do you have a smoker's cough?" Often the reply is, "No way. I would stop smoking if I did." But a cough isn't a disease, it's another of nature's survival techniques to eject harmful deposits from our lungs. Vomiting is another survival technique to eject poisons from our stomachs.

Taking a drug means that you are altering the calibration of one or more of your senses – the instruments on which your wellbeing depends. The increased security, courage, confidence and happiness we experience when we free ourselves from addiction is truly priceless.

But we are more than mere machines run by computers. The resourcefulness of the human spirit is phenomenal. Look around you. Every single day, so-called 'ordinary' people act with astonishing heroism and they're not using cannabis to do it.

A huge number of US military service people returned home from the Vietnam War in the 1970s after extensively using cannabis, cocaine, LSD, heroin and other drugs for the duration of their service there. They were seriously addicted to the drugs. Hundreds of thousands of them.

Yet studies concluded that more than 90 per cent got free from the addiction overnight. Without any problems at all. With hardly any, if any, support at all. With professional support, that percentage would doubtless have been even higher.

You're about to be set free overnight too. Easily, without any pain and without feeling any sense of loss.

WILL I BE ABLE TO ENJOY
LIFE AFTER I QUIT?

That's the question that puts a lot of addicts off even trying to quit. As with all addictions, it's not just where you are going to that is so important, it's what you are escaping from that counts.

All those doped-up days and nights out? There is something that beats them hands down. Partying and dancing all night with friends without the need or desire to consume an addictive, toxic substance that regularly makes you feel moody, anxious, paranoid, sad, terrified, ashamed and regretful.

Freedom from a drug that makes you feel lousy and controls you while costing you a fortune.

The real pleasure in those good-time situations always came from the company of your friends, the party atmosphere and the dancing. You can carry on with all that, with beautiful abandon.

From here on it's all guilt free. It's all fun.

Cannabis has been cadging a ride on the back of these genuine pleasures. Now you can be a party animal without the need for any drugs.

That said, you'll probably be amazed how many dull, drab, boring events and people you can happily choose to avoid after you quit. All those places and people you sought out simply to feed your addiction? You won't need them any more. You'll get your choice back.

IS IT REALLY POSSIBLE TO QUIT FOREVER?

Disregard what other so-called experts tell you about addiction. They may mean well but they are unwittingly adding to the fear and confusion surrounding the subject. Addiction is not an all-powerful, mystical phenomenon or a permanent illness or condition that you can never free yourself from. At its root is a simple misunderstanding. Your brain mistakes the drug as the thing that provides relief from cannabis withdrawal, when, in fact, it's the cause of it.

This back-to-front thinking allows the brainwashing to take root and grow in your mind. That is the illusion that cannabis provides you with a genuine pleasure or crutch. This leads to a feeling of deprivation when you try to cut down or quit.

I once said to someone I was helping get free from drugs, "Why don't you just think of yourself as someone who, by definition, under no circumstances ever takes drugs and get on with your life?"

Imagine being in a place whereby you could do that. Well, you're very nearly there. And far from feeling a sense of sacrifice or regret or loss, when you are finally free from cannabis you'll be barely able to resist shouting from the rooftops about how happy you are. Whether you've been smoking dope for just a few years or you've been addicted to cannabis for decades, this method will set you free.

If you haven't lost everyone and everything already, good on you. You're about to get out just in time. If, on the other hand, you're on your own, alone, already having lost it all, don't worry.

"IT'S NEVER TOO LATE TO GET YOUR LIFE BACK."

By the way, those are the words of one of our recent clients, not our own. Whatever your history with cannabis, the future is all of a sudden looking extremely bright for you.

Chapter 10

GETTING FREE

How many times have you gone without things you or your family need just so you could buy dope? It's bad enough when it's life's little luxuries that they've had to go without – it's sadder still when it's life's essentials.

No doubt there have been times when you've got so upset with yourself about your cannabis use that you've felt ashamed and useless, right down at rock bottom, and you've said, "Never again. I simply can't do this anymore." And you may have cried and felt ashamed and curled up in your bed.

But what happened a week later? Or a few weeks later? Despite all that anguish, you were back on it, believing escape was impossible.

Start seeing your addiction like that white chalk circle. You can step outside it forever any time you want to. We're good at seeing other people's white chalk circles for what they are but we need our own chalk circles to be pointed out to us. It's time to start seeing your own for what it is.

We've established that, as drug addicts, we completely overestimate the things we think the drug does for us.

With cannabis, we're fooled into thinking it relaxes us or makes us more creative and interesting and confident. In fact, it does none of those things. In your heart, at this moment, you know it does the complete opposite. Look at your life. In how many ways has the drug led you to this point, seeking help to get free?

See the drug as it really is. Acknowledge how you became brainwashed and conned into believing it gave you some kind of pleasure or benefit. Understand and accept that withdrawal pangs are very mild and barely noticeable. There is no danger whatsoever, nor anything to fear. Cannabis withdraws from the body incredibly quickly. In just three to five days, you won't even notice it.

Any unpleasantness is created by what's in your mind. Get your mindset right, understand that you're not giving up anything, and quitting will be easy.

YOU'RE NOT STUCK WITH CANNABIS

Anyone can quit. Your chances of quitting are not governed by your personality or your DNA or any other preset condition. You're not stuck in this trap because you're stupid or weak. Highly intelligent people seek the help of Easyway all the time. Just like you, the addiction convinced them that cannabis played a part in their success. They seek our help when they realise it's beginning to dismantle it.

They realise that, rather than giving them inspiration or stress relief, it does the opposite; rather than giving their personality a lift, it makes them arrogant and boring; and where they thought they were in control of it, they now realise it's controlling them.

The classic American novel *Of Mice and Men* by John Steinbeck features a relationship which could equally be our relationship with drug addiction. Lenny worships George, partly because George saved him from drowning in a river. Poor Lenny is so slow and mentally challenged that he entirely disregards the fact that it was George who pushed him to go into the river in the first place, in the full knowledge that he couldn't swim and would certainly drown if not rescued. Nevertheless, Lenny remains blindly grateful to George in spite of the facts.

No matter how low the drug drags us down, we remain grateful for the perceived pleasures that we're conned into believing it provides.

We end up in a triple low: 1. the very slight physical withdrawal; 2. the mental craving that is triggered by that, making you feel constantly aggravated, deprived and miserable; and 3. on top of that the drug drags your body, mind and spirit to greater and greater depths, destroying relationships, careers and friendships. And all of that – the constant state of misery and dissatisfaction – ends up feeling like NORMAL. Imagine how great you'll feel when you get rid of the dope and return to your genuine state of normality; calm, satisfied, relaxed, and content.

REMEMBER, CANNABIS DOESN'T FIX THE MISERY AND DISSATISFACTION, IT CAUSES IT.

When we try to quit with the wrong method the experience does us tremendous harm, driving us deeper into the trap. At Narcotics Anonymous the first thing we're told is that we're powerless over our addiction. Great! We're basically told to surrender to the addiction and acknowledge that we have two options: a lifelong struggle or submission to the drug.

That's the same as telling someone who thinks they're trapped inside a white circle of chalk that they can't move out of that circle – they're trapped. We don't need to take 12 steps, we just need to take the one – simply stepping across the white chalk line.

You can believe you have an addictive personality if you want to, it really doesn't matter. Follow this method and you will still find it easy to stop... permanently.

The theory of addictive personality or genes stems from looking at the situation from the wrong perspective. It's not your personality or genes that gets you addicted, it's your belief that you get some kind of pleasure or crutch from the drug.

You got hooked on cannabis because you took some, simple as that. Taking the drug is what triggers the cycle of addiction. Say you were proven to have an addictive personality but never took the drug in your life: do you think you would be addicted? Cannabis is addictive and people without addictive personalities or genes, if such things exist, get addicted to it too. The way out is the same for everyone, regardless of your genes or personality. And it's easy.

STOP TAKING THE DRUG.

FORGET CUTTING DOWN

Remember that the way addiction works is completely in conflict with restricting your intake to a limited amount. Addiction compels us to take more and more. By cutting down, you commit to a life of inner conflict, deprivation, frustration and ultimate failure. What about all the people who seem to get away with only having a joint every now and then? Don't envy them after today. They're all putting on a brave face or playing with fire.

There are a few different types. Firstly, the outright liars. They'll tell you they only ever have a joint or two a month and never feel inclined to have more. Yet you notice they're always having a joint whenever you see them. They lie to you and to themselves.

Then there are the very occasional users. They barely ever have a joint. If nothing else they prove how weak the addiction is because they go through complete withdrawal every time they take dope. Often, if they're honest, they don't even think they're enjoying the experience – they don't particularly like the taste, the smell or even feeling high, so it puts them off for another six months.

They're playing with fire, though, because that's how most addicts start out. They're the fly at the top of the pitcher plant and all it needs is something to change in their life – hitting a bad patch – for them to fall all the way in.

Then there are the apparently moderate users. Often, like the liars, they normally have more of it, more often than they're prepared to admit. Some of them, though, simply can't cope with more of the poison. Their bodies aren't strong enough. Some can't work efficiently if they have too much of the drug and others are protective of their careers. They don't want to lose their job for failing a random drug test.

Whatever their motivation, it forces them to limit the amount of dope they take. It's like being on a permanent diet. They wait days and days until they allow themselves to finally have a joint and then they have another and another. The longer they wait between uses, the more precious it seems to be when they finally cave in.

That's why cutting down doesn't work. That plus the fact that addiction simply doesn't ever get less severe. The only way out is to kill the Little Monster by quitting completely.

DIFFICULT CIRCUMSTANCES

Some people say the reason they got hooked is because they have or had deep-rooted issues in their life. With all respect, this is another red herring.

Many people are born into incredibly difficult and challenging lives. Not all of them become drug addicts. But because of the brainwashing that tells us drugs are a kind of "cure-all" that can lift you out of your grim reality, people who have suffered bad experiences on a long-term basis might be more likely to take drugs. Even so, that doesn't make it harder for them to get free.

The simple belief that they're particularly badly addicted or prone to be addicted because of their circumstances easily turns into one of those white chalk circles. It's based on the exact same nonsense. It's as easy for them, as for anyone, to step out of the circle and set themselves free. They just have to use the right method.

Let's examine this argument a little more.

Are there people with deep-rooted issues who smoke dope?

Yes.

Are there people with deep-rooted issues who have never once smoked dope?

Yes.

Are there people without deep-rooted issues whose only real problem in life is that they're addicted to cannabis?

Yes.

Are there people without deep-rooted issues who don't have a cannabis problem?

Yes.

Can you see how there is no connection whatsoever? Now someone who has deep-rooted issues may well also have a cannabis problem but the deep-rooted issues are not the cause of the cannabis problem. If they were, everyone with a deep-rooted problem would take cannabis and no-one without deep-rooted issues would become addicted.

Imagine you have a spot on your face. Someone gives you an ointment that they say will clear it up. You rub it onto the spot and it magically disappears.

A week later the spot returns, bigger and redder this time. You apply more of the ointment and it disappears again. Five days later the spot returns, but now it's more than just a spot, it's a rash. As time goes on, the gap between the rash of spots breaking out becomes shorter and the rash of spots gets bigger and bigger and itchier and itchier each time.

Imagine the horror you would feel as you realised that it's just going to get worse and worse unless you find a cure. Imagine you've become so reliant on that ointment that you're prepared to pay a fortune for it and you have to take it everywhere with you, because you're afraid the rash could break out at any time.

Then you discover that you're not alone, there are millions of other people suffering with the exact same problem and they're all handing over a fortune to the ointment industry.

The nightmare goes on and on. Then one day you meet a man who says he used to have the exact same problem but solved it. You ask him his secret and he tells you.

STOP USING THE OINTMENT.

He advises you to do the same and reassures you that the rash and spots will clear up in a matter of days, after which:

YOU WILL NEVER SUFFER IT AGAIN.

What would you do? Would you feel miserable that you could never use the ointment again? Or would you be elated that you'll never have to?

Now apply this logic to cannabis. You have the power to free yourself. How amazing is that?

Chapter 11

THE SIXTH INSTRUCTION

We want you to make an informed decision to get rid of cannabis. Over time you'll notice some wonderful changes taking place. Your bank balance will look healthier. You'll look and feel a whole lot better – your "Normal" having been raised back up from that triple low. You'll realise how much energy and vitality the drug stole from you.

At those moments, remind yourself that you're enjoying normality. There's nothing special about it. It's what you've escaped from that's really important. Always look back and smile about what you've left behind.

The sixth instruction is designed to help you with this:

MAKE A WRITTEN RECORD OF HOW CANNABIS AFFECTED YOUR LIFE.

Write down what life was like for you as a dope addict. What was it about that life that made you want to quit?

Make sure you write it in the past tense. This is what you have escaped from, remember, not where you're going.

Don't hold back on the detail. For example, you could say, "Life as a dope addict made me feel unhealthy," but it is more useful to paint a fuller picture: "Life as a dope addict messed with my body, my mind and my spirit. I felt constantly tired, on edge and horribly unhealthy. That made me feel miserable and wretched." It is important that you include details of the factors and how they made you feel – all in the past tense.

The above is just an example. Make it personal to you, in your own words, describing your own feelings. Do this with all the aspects of your life as a dope addict. For example, you could say, "It controlled my life, what I did, when I did it and how I felt when I was doing it and that made me feel weak."

Once you've done that for every aspect of your life as a dope addict, carry that record with you wherever you go, because I'd like you to refer to it at certain times. Be comfortable with the knowledge that you are going to think about cannabis from time to time, even though you probably feel worried that you might think about it too much. It's worrying about it that is the problem. If you try not to think about cannabis, you will think about it even more. Remember that elephant we spoke about?

Cast your mind back to the I Want A Joint diagram in Chapter 7. It's not a problem if you think about cannabis from time to time, even if you think, "I WANT A JOINT." That's just an echo from the routines that you associated with your dope taking. It's very easy to remind yourself that you're free from all that and rejoice in the knowledge that you no longer need the drug.

Some people find this difficult to accept but it is true. Think about it. If you were arguing with a friend or lover, at the height of the argument you might think, "I COULD KILL YOU NOW," but it doesn't mean you could, does it? It doesn't make you a killer. It's just a thought and it's what you do with the thought that matters.

Say you parked your car in the same parking space every day for a year. Then one day your parking space was moved one space down. It wouldn't be a big surprise if you parked in the old parking space by mistake, would it? But how would you react? Would you turn the engine off, throw your hands in the air and think to yourself, "Damn, I'm infatuated with this parking space! I'm emotionally attached to it. I can't possibly park my car in the new space." Or would you just smile to yourself and move your car?

Automatically following old habits and routines isn't a sign that you want that old routine back. It just means that your brain has momentarily forgotten that there has been a change. So if, after you've quit, the thought of taking cannabis comes into your mind, it doesn't mean the Little Monster is winning or that you need to fight anything, it's just a sign that your brain has forgotten that you're no longer hooked. And every time you remember it's a marvellous moment.

Rather than worrying about it, or panicking about it, or trying not to think about it, welcome the thought and say to yourself,

"GREAT, I'M FREE!"

And feel good about it. If you need a nudge in the right direction this is an excellent time to read your record of what life was like for you as an addict. So put the book down now and write that record. It only needs to be a page long. Then carry it with you. It's a wonderful written testimony of what you're escaping from.

We need these reminders because it's amazing how quickly the body and brain forget pain. It's actually part of our survival mechanism. If you could recollect pain and misery exactly how they were at the time, you'd be doubled up in pain every time you remembered the time you broke your leg, or the time you banged your head on a low beam. For this reason the brain filters out and dilutes memory of pain or painful incidents. Be aware of this because once you've quit, something might happen that reminds you about cannabis or triggers a rose-tinted memory of how life used to be on the drug – a phoney memory, which overlooks how bad you really felt. This is where the written record proves invaluable.

Chapter 12

REGAINING CONTROL

Those who consider themselves in control of their cannabis use suffer the illusion of pleasure more than those who realise that they've lost control. But ask them to define the pleasure and they can't give a convincing reason for taking the drug. Instead, they offer defensive excuses:

"I can take it or leave it."

"I don't do it that much."

"It's not doing me any harm."

If you genuinely enjoy something, why would you choose to leave it? The only possible reason is that you know it's causing a problem. If you didn't think it was a problem and you genuinely enjoyed it, why go without for any length of time?

If a friend told you that they love bananas but only have one once a month, would you think, "There's someone who's in control of their bananas"? Or would you think, "Wow! I didn't know she had a banana problem."

As for the argument, "It's not doing me any harm," besides the fact that we all know it's untrue, is it any reason for doing something? Wearing a top hat and singing "Waltzing Matilda" doesn't do any harm, but that's not enough of a reason to make anyone do it.

BURNING QUESTIONS

You are entering the exciting final stages before becoming a non-dope addict, but you may still have some lingering concerns. So let's remove any traces of uncertainty.

Right now you should be feeling like a parachutist about to make a jump. You've been through proper instruction, you've paid attention and understood how it all works and you have complete faith in what you're about to do.

You're about to experience an exhilarating sense of freedom. That's what you were hoping for when you boarded the plane and that's what you've been prepared for. You should feel confident about your every move.

But it's completely understandable that, as you stand by the door of the plane, looking out at this wonderful new experience that awaits you, you feel the butterflies in your stomach and a little knot of apprehension. Those butterflies are completely natural and while you can tell yourself that there is no rational reason for feeling apprehensive, it is the natural human response when facing something new, even when that experience could be the best thing that's ever happened to you.

Before they finish off the Big Monster, cannabis addicts fear that, although they wish they didn't take it, they will have to go through some terrible ordeal in order to quit, or that life will never be enjoyable again without the drug. Even though they know that it's making them miserable, these fears cause them to put off what they see as the evil day. We've all said it:

"I will stop, just not right now."

It's no surprise that we have these fears. All our lives we are led to believe that dope provides tremendous pleasure and support and that addictions are incurable. Yet we're convinced that we won't get hooked. These myths are ingrained among our beliefs before we even have our first joint. No wonder we find it difficult to believe that stopping can be easy.

THE MOMENT OF REVELATION

You deserve a pat on the back for following the instructions this far and making a positive move to end your dope problem. You'll be eager to get to the end and experience that exhilarating sense of freedom that you've been promised, but you may be wondering when exactly does that moment come?

How will you know when you're truly free from cannabis addiction?

- When you can go a whole day without a joint?
- When you can go a week?
- When you can enjoy social events without cannabis?

In fact, it's none of the above. Unlike other methods, with Easyway you don't have to wait to experience that glorious certainty that you're free.

YOU KNOW YOU'VE QUIT WHEN YOU NO LONGER FEEL ANY NEED OR DESIRE TO TAKE CANNABIS.

Waiting to reach a given milestone assumes that you'll start off with a feeling of sacrifice or deprivation and hope it will fade over time. If you do that, the feeling of deprivation will only grow over time and you'll be left wondering indefinitely whether you've succeeded or not. You'll be in the absurd position of waiting for something *not* to happen.

It's not the joint you *think* will be your last, or the one you *hope* will be your last; when you quit with Easyway there is no doubt. You know – and it's a marvellous feeling.

The only way you might regard your final joint with uncertainty is if you use the willpower method, or, for some reason, you fail to follow all the instructions. Be absolutely clear about this: you will not miss dope and you will enjoy life more and be better equipped to cope with stress when you're free.

YOU HAVE EVERYTHING TO GAIN.

People who quit with the willpower method spend their time suspecting that there could be bad news lurking just around the corner. It's like a dark shadow stalking their every move. They are on the lookout for a sign that their attempt to quit has failed. Imagine living the rest of your life like that – hoping you're free but not being convinced and worrying that the misery and degradation could return at any moment.

This is why the willpower method makes people so miserable. They have to endure the rest of their lives waiting for nothing to happen. It's hardly surprising the vast majority fail.

THE REMOVAL OF DOUBT

Some people reach this stage of the book convinced that they understand everything and are ready to quit. If that's you, fantastic, but let's not jump the gun. If it's not you and you haven't yet achieved that certainty, don't worry, all will become clear. Whatever your current level of certainty, please take the time and care to pay attention right to the end of the book. You're very nearly there.

It's perfectly understandable that so many dope addicts believe that stopping will be incredibly hard. There is nothing stupid or unusual in that belief. We're subjected to this misinformation all our lives and then we reinforce it by trying to quit with the willpower method. All your failed attempts to quit or cut down simply serve to reinforce the belief that stopping requires a superhuman effort.

That desperate craving you get when you're fighting the desire to have a joint may conflict with everything you know about the evils of the drug but the craving is still very real and so is the irritability and misery you feel when you use willpower to try to stop.

Addiction puts us in a state of confusion. When we're forced to consider cannabis logically, we can see clearly that it's a mug's game, yet we still feel a desire to do it and this creates an inner tension. The fact that we can't put our finger on what precise pleasure the drug gives us only serves to increase the confusion. We can't define it but we assume there must be some pleasure or benefit, otherwise why keep taking it?

Remember these facts:

- The desire to take cannabis comes from the Big Monster – the illusion that the drug gives us pleasure or support.
- The edgy feeling we get when we're without dope is merely the Little Monster wanting to be fed.
- The Little Monster was created by taking dope in the first place.
- Therefore, taking dope does not relieve the anxiety, it causes it.

Once you have these facts clearly established in your mind, it's easy to see that if you remove the cause of the anxiety you will immediately start to enjoy life free from the drug.

The willpower method is all about fighting through the anxiety; with Easyway you remove it altogether. In the first few days after quitting with the willpower method, when your will is at its strongest, you may have the upper hand in the battle. But over time your resolve is likely to weaken, the uncertainty sets in and the craving increases.

Now your mind is torn in two, one half determined to be a non-dope addict, the other urging you to carry on. Is it surprising that we get so confused, irritable and miserable on the willpower method? It would be a miracle if we didn't!

Even if you starve the Little Monster to death, without destroying the Big Monster you will remain forever vulnerable to the temptation to use dope again. With Easyway, you kill the Big Monster first. You unravel the brainwashing and see the drug for what it really is: an addictive poison that controls and debilitates those who take it. Then the Little Monster is easy to deal with. In fact, you can enjoy the process, confident in the knowledge that you're destroying a mortal enemy.

REMOVING TEMPTATION

Unless you destroy the Big Monster – the brainwashing that creates the desire to take cannabis – you always remain vulnerable to temptation. So when Narcotics Anonymous tells its clients they're never cured from addiction, they're right. With the willpower method it's true. As long as the temptation remains, there will always be the danger of slipping back into the trap.

AA and NA do amazing work all over the world and the last thing we'd want to do is knock them, particularly as they've helped so many people, but this way, Easyway, is different. A question we're often asked is, "Once I'm cured, will I be able to have the odd joint?"

The answer is simple: "Once you're cured, why would you want to?"

If you approach your final joint still thinking that the odd puff now and again would be nice, you haven't followed all the instructions and the Big Monster still lurks in your mind.

There will be times when you're tested. Other dope users who don't understand the addiction trap will see how confident and in control you are as a non-addict and will assume the one joint won't set you back. What these dope addicts don't understand is that you have absolutely no desire to have just the one. But you understand it.

With the willpower method, you're told that one joint is all it will take to drag you back into the pit. Here NA is correct again. The point is that with Easyway, you no longer have any desire to have "just one joint" than you do to take cyanide.

LIVING LIFE TO THE FULL

As addicts we fear that if we take dope out of our lives we will take out the enjoyment too. It's easy to see why such a belief would stop anyone from trying to quit. But the truth is, cannabis and other addictive drugs actually reduce your ability to derive genuine enjoyment or excitement from anything in life. Drugs debilitate your senses, play havoc with your judgement, make you crushingly dull, vulnerable and insecure and often result in you feeling sick, guilty and full of remorse.

The brainwashing creates a romanticised image of taking dope. Where you have had good times involving the drug, a quick analysis of all the details of those times will reveal that there were other factors that made them enjoyable: good company, good food, beautiful setting, great entertainment, a happy occasion...

If you can think of occasions like this that you consider to have been enjoyable because you were taking dope, consider them carefully and try to understand why the dope appeared to enhance the situation. It doesn't take much to see that in reality it does the opposite.

Rather than holding on to the illusion that such occasions won't be enjoyable again without dope, remind yourself that you will now be able to enjoy those occasions more because you'll be free from three tyrants: the debilitating effects of addiction, the lethargy, anxiety and guilt that come with dope, and the sheer misery of knowing you're an addict.

Most of the time we're not even aware of how dope makes us feel. The only time we're really aware of it is when we want to have it but can't, or we're taking it but wishing we didn't have to.

THROW AWAY THE ROTTEN CRUTCH

The cannabis myth doesn't just make us believe we get pleasure from the drug, it also convinces us that we derive some kind of support from the drug – as if life would be unmanageable without it! Of course, this is the complete opposite of the truth, yet as dope addicts we believe it and tend to turn to our drug in times of stress.

There are many stressful situations in life: a family row, pressure at work, financial worries or just feeling you need to let your hair down. As a dope addict you take yourself away, get stoned and put your problems out of your mind.

But sooner or later you have to return to the real world and, surprise, surprise, the problems are still there. In fact, they've usually got worse. If you continue to believe that dope is your little crutch to lean on in these stressful situations, what will happen the next time such a situation arises after you've quit? Your brain will tell you, "At times like this I would have had a spliff." And you'll feel deprived that you can no longer do so.

Be honest, have you ever found yourself in the middle of a domestic row and thought, "It doesn't matter that we're shouting horrible things at one another and it's really painful because I can just go and get stoned and it will be all right"? Or did the fact that you do dope make the row worse?

Non-dope addicts also have to deal with stress but they're not left moping because they can't have dope. All you have to do is accept that, like all non-addicts, you will have ups and downs in your life after you've quit and understand that if you start wishing you could do dope in such situations, you will be moping for an illusion and creating a void.

If you can anticipate the difficult times in life after you've quit and prepare yourself mentally for them, you won't get caught out. Remind yourself that any stress you feel is not because you can't have cannabis. In fact, taking cannabis would only make it worse. Much worse.

If you think about cannabis when life gets stressful, use that thought to remind yourself that you're free, no longer a miserable slave, and your endless downward spiral into the pit of addiction is over. Use that thought and rejoice.

Chapter 13

REMOVING FEAR

Your release from the cannabis trap is imminent, so let's make sure you have established a positive, excited mindset.

Sadly, there is a common phenomenon among convicts of reoffending soon after they are released from prison. This isn't because they're stupid and believe they can get away with it this time, it's because they're frightened by the unfamiliarity of life on the outside and crave the 'security' of jail. It's what they know.

If you happened to know an ex-con like that, who was struggling to believe that he could cope with life outside prison, wouldn't you want to help by showing him how much better life is when you're free? You'd point out all the wonderful things you can do, at your leisure, not when you're permitted to do them. Things like:

• Seeing friends
• Going for a walk in the park
• Taking a trip somewhere
• Having a nice meal in a restaurant or a picnic in the park

• Going to the cinema or theatre
• Having a lie-in with your lover

Of course, the ex-con would know all these things but he might have lost sight of just how enjoyable they are. When you're in prison and denied the usual pleasures in life, your idea of pleasure changes.

The cannabis trap is a prison. When you're addicted you lose the ability to enjoy the things you enjoyed before you started taking it. The drug-induced illusion of pleasure takes the place of genuine pleasures and becomes the thing you live for. But it's an illusion.

AS AN ADDICT YOU SPEND YOUR LIFE CHASING AN ILLUSION, CONSTANTLY TRYING TO ESCAPE FROM A LOW.

The genuine pleasures still exist and they're still enjoyable, but when all you want is dope, they don't seem appealing to you. If you knew an ex-con who was struggling to see this and risking his freedom as a result, wouldn't you do everything in your power to make him see things as they really are?

If you can do that for someone else, why not do it for yourself? Think about all the pleasures that you have enjoyed in your life without cannabis and start looking forward to enjoying those pleasures again. It will help if you write them down. Your list may have a similar look to the example above for the ex-con and the more you think about it, the more you will add to it. Take your time. What is important is that you establish the right frame of mind to quit with a feeling of excitement and certainty.

WHAT YOU'VE ACHIEVED SO FAR

In Chapter 1 I explained how Easyway works like the combination to a safe. For it to work you need to know all the numbers and apply them in the correct order. You may have found that frustrating at the time. That's understandable. You were eager to discover the cure to your problem and probably wondered why we couldn't just reveal the secret at the start.

By now you should understand why that is not possible. You have to follow the instructions in the correct order for the method to work and the Big Monster to be conquered. If you have done that, you now stand on the brink of becoming a happy non-addict. You have come a long way towards achieving the state of mind necessary for you to quit and remain free for the rest of your life.

Congratulations! That is some achievement. Remember how you used to think quitting was virtually impossible, that there would be a painful withdrawal process, that you would feel miserable and deprived, and that the temptation to smoke dope would always be nagging away at you?

Well, now you know that's not the case. You have every reason to feel excited. You're setting yourself free from a prison that has brought you nothing but misery and stress and you're choosing a life that will bring you a happiness you may have forgotten even existed.

Perhaps you think that's an exaggeration and that you have no reason to congratulate yourself. You may have changed your mindset and feel confident that you can stop, but you're still not convinced that being a non-dope addict will be the wonderful experience we make it out to be.

It's time to address the fear of success.

THE FEAR OF SUCCESS

The fear of life outside jail can keep the prisoner in the trap. He feels secure in his prison because it's an environment he knows. Even though it's a life of confinement and austerity, he fears it less than the world outside, which is alien and riddled with uncertainty.

When we relate this fear to quitting cannabis, we have established that the fear is caused by illusions. These illusions have been put in your brain by many influences, some of which are well-meaning but misguided, some have a vested interest in you continuing to be addicted to cannabis. You've been brainwashed into believing that cannabis gives you some sort of pleasure or support.

You're also afraid that the process of stopping will be an ordeal that you will not be able to bear for long enough to succeed. With Easyway you succeed in becoming a non-cannabis addict the moment you finish your final joint and feel no desire ever to take the drug again.

Some people see the cannabis trap as a hole in the ground: something you fall into easily but struggle to get out of. But that's not the case. Though it may feel like a deep, dark hole you're in, there's no physical effort required to escape. You simply need to make a choice. It's a simple choice between taking a step backwards or a step forward.

You can either choose to remain in the trap for the rest of your life, becoming more and more enslaved and miserable, or you can choose the opposite. There is no benefit whatsoever to being in the cannabis trap. You were lured into it by a set of illusions that bombarded you from a young age. And you've found that it makes you miserable.

SO NOW YOU JUST HAVE TO MAKE A SIMPLE CHOICE. TAKE A STEP FORWARDS.

It's as simple as that. The fear of success can only stop you if you continue to believe that you get some pleasure or support from the drug.

The fears that serve us well are instinctive. For example, the fear of heights, fire or the sea are natural responses that protect us from falling, getting burned or drowning. There's nothing instinctive about the fear of escaping from the cannabis trap.

YOU HAVE NOTHING TO FEAR

Once you're free from the trap, you'll be amazed at how easy it was to escape. You'll find that you're able to derive far more pleasure from life and your only reason for regret will be not having made your escape sooner. At the moment you may still feel like someone struggling to get out of a deep pit, but once you do get out you'll realise your fears were groundless.

In order to achieve this success you need to clear your mind of all doubt. Understand and accept that your fears of trying to live without cannabis are based on illusions. Remind yourself what those illusions are and how your experience, when you stop to think, has proven them all to have no validity whatsoever.

Do this and you'll quickly see that, in reality, you have nothing to fear.

On the subject of falling back into the trap, some people ask, "How can you know for certain that something will not happen?" In other words, even if you do manage to quit cannabis, how do you know you won't get hooked again? After all, nothing is one hundred per cent certain, is it?

Actually, it is when it's in your control. Once you've seen through the confidence trick that lured you into the trap in the first place, you will have no difficulty in deciding to stay free. And if that's your decision, it will happen. If you still have doubts and fears at this stage, don't worry, that's not at all unusual. You've been brainwashed into thinking you have to go through some painful ordeal and make huge sacrifices to become a non-dope addict and that even if you do succeed, you will be forever tempted to take dope.

Recognising and accepting this is not the case is purely a matter of changing the way you look at the situation. Once you're in the right frame of mind, you will change your perception and the fear will go.

The fifth instruction was to keep an open mind. If you've followed this instruction, you'll have seen through the illusions to the true picture: that cannabis does absolutely nothing for you whatsoever. It's neither a source of pleasure nor support; in fact, it takes away genuine pleasures and leaves you feeling vulnerable.

If you're still unclear on this point, go back and read Chapter 3 again, making sure you allow your mind to take it all on board. Relax, let go of your preconceptions and allow the true picture to take shape in your mind.

The key to seeing through any illusion is not through willpower, it's through letting go of your existing perceptions and allowing your mind to see it another way.

Chapter 14

FIRST STEPS TO FREEDOM

You've made great progress already in the process of unravelling the brainwashing that has kept you hooked on cannabis and you should be aware of achieving the right frame of mind to escape. The Big Monster is being destroyed.

Now it's time to start taking the practical forward steps that will see you become a happy non-addict for the rest of your life. Your first positive step was choosing to read this book. And you did have a choice in that: you could have continued to bury your head in the sand and stumble further and further into the miserable slavery of addiction. Instead you decided to take positive action to resolve the situation.

Keep making those positive choices.

As we move forward, there are three very important facts that you need to remember:

1. CANNABIS DOES ABSOLUTELY NOTHING FOR YOU AT ALL.

It's crucial that you understand why this is true and accept it to be the case, so that you never get a feeling of deprivation or sacrifice.

2. THERE IS NO NEED FOR A TRANSITIONAL PERIOD.

Anyone who quits with Easyway has no need to worry about the withdrawal period. Yes, it may take time to repair the physical damage caused by drug, but the moment you stop taking it is the moment you become free. You don't have to wait for anything to happen.

3. THERE IS NO SUCH THING AS "JUST THE ONE".

Just one joint – in fact, just one puff of one joint – is enough to make you a cannabis addict again and must be seen for what it is: part of a lifelong chain of self-destruction. If you can see that there is no benefit in taking cannabis you will have no desire to do so, not even "just the one".

KILL THE BIG MONSTER

It's a stark indication of just how severely the brainwashing distorts our perceptions that anyone should come to regard a drug that is destroying them and making them miserable as their friend and support.

Yet countless addicts are taken in by the myth that they can never get completely free. They fear that if they quit they will not only lose their closest companion, they will lose a part of themselves.

If you've ever lost a genuine friend, you'll know the feeling of real grief. Eventually you come to terms with the loss and life goes on, but it leaves a void in your life that you can never fill. Still, there's nothing you can do about it. You have no choice but to accept the situation and, though it still hurts, you do.

When drug addicts try to quit through willpower, they too feel they're losing a friend. They know that they're making the right decision to stop, but they feel they're making a sacrifice and that creates a void in their lives. Unlike real grief, it isn't a genuine void, but they believe it is and so the effect is the same. They feel as if they're mourning for a friend.

But wait! This false friend isn't even dead. The drugs are always there, luring the addict back in.

There should be no confusion between quitting cannabis and losing a friend. Cannabis is a tyrant that has held you captive, made your life miserable, robbed you of time, money, relationships perhaps, and tried to convince you that there is no escape. Imagine if you lived under such a tyrant and then the tyrant died. Would you mourn? No, you would rejoice.

When you kill the Big Monster, you can rejoice and celebrate straight away and you can continue to rejoice and celebrate for the rest of your life.

GET IT CLEAR IN YOUR MIND THAT CANNABIS NEVER WAS AND NEVER WILL BE YOUR FRIEND.

Nor is it part of your identity. It never has been, and by getting rid of it, you're sacrificing nothing, just making marvellous, positive gains.

So the answer to the question, "When will I be free?" is, "Whenever you choose to be." You could spend the next few days, and possibly the rest of your life, continuing to believe that cannabis was your friend and wondering when you'll stop missing it. If so, you'll feel miserable, the desire to take cannabis may never leave you and you'll either end up feeling deprived for the rest of your life or you'll end up going back to cannabis and feeling even worse.

Alternatively, you can recognise the drug for the mortal enemy that it really is and take pleasure in cutting it out of your life. Then you need never crave it again and whenever it enters your mind you'll feel elated that it's no longer destroying you.

Unlike people who quit with the willpower method, you'll be happy to think about your old enemy and you needn't try to block it from your mind. On the contrary, enjoy thinking about it and rejoice that it no longer plagues your life.

KILL THE LITTLE MONSTER

During the first few days after your final joint, the Little Monster may be grumbling away, sending messages to your brain that it wants you to interpret as, "I want a joint." But you now understand the true picture and, instead of doing dope, or getting into a panic because you can't, pause for a moment. Take a deep breath. Remind yourself there is nothing to fear. There is no pain. The feeling isn't bad. It's just the slight uncomfortable feeling that occurs when cannabis leaves your system.

It's what dope addicts suffer throughout their addicted lives.

Before you started this book your mind interpreted the pangs of the Little Monster as "I want a joint" because it had every reason to believe that cannabis would satisfy the empty, insecure feeling. But now, having killed the Big Monster, you understand that, far from relieving that feeling, it's cannabis that caused it.

So relax, accept the feeling for what it really is – the death throes of the Little Monster – and remind yourself, "Non-dope addicts don't have this problem.

This is a feeling that addicts suffer and they suffer it throughout their addicted lives. Isn't it great?! It will soon be gone forever."

The withdrawal pangs will cease to feel like pangs and will become moments of pleasure.

During the first few days in particular you might find that you forget you've quit. It can happen at any time. You think, "I'll have a joint," and then you remember with joy that you're now a non-dope addict. But you wonder why the thought entered your head when you were convinced you'd reversed the brainwashing.

Such times can be crucial in whether you succeed or not. React in the wrong way and they can set you right back. Doubts can surface and you may start to question your decision to quit and lose faith in yourself.

These situations won't catch you out if you're ready for them. Prepare yourself mentally so that when they occur you remain calm and use them as a reminder of the wonderful freedom you've gained. Instead of thinking, "I can't do this," you will think, "Isn't it great?! I don't need to take cannabis any more. I'm free!"

Be aware too that the associations you used to make with taking cannabis, such as seeing friends, eating out, going to parties etc, can linger on after the Little Monster has died. For dope addicts who quit with the willpower method, this can seriously undermine their efforts. In their minds they have built up a powerful case against cannabis, they've decided to become a non-addict, they've managed to go for however long without any of the drug and yet, on certain occasions, a voice keeps saying, "I want a joint."

The problem is they haven't killed the Big Monster, so they still think of cannabis as a pleasure or support.

Although you will no longer suffer the illusion that you're being deprived, it's still vital that you prepare yourself for these situations. Occasionally forgetting that you no longer take cannabis isn't a bad sign, it's a very good one. It's proof that your life is returning to the happy state you were in before you got hooked, when your whole existence wasn't dominated by a poisonous and highly addictive drug.

Remember the parking space analogy. Thoughts don't matter – it's what you do with the thoughts that matters.

Expecting these moments to happen and being prepared for them will save you from being caught off guard. You'll be wearing a suit of impregnable armour. You know you've made the correct decision and nobody will be able to make you doubt it. Instead of being the cause of your downfall, these moments will give you added strength and pleasure, reminding you just how wonderful it is to be FREE!

SHED YOUR CANNABIS SKIN

Everything you've read so far was designed to help you understand the trap you're in and recognise that you hold the key to get out. The trap is the addiction. The key is unravelling the brainwashing that keeps you addicted – killing the Big Monster. The final step is to turn the key – to kill the Little Monster – and walk free.

You should be completely clear how the cannabis trap keeps you hooked by creating the illusion of pleasure. You should understand that any benefit you thought you got from cannabis was merely an illusion created by a combination of the Little and Big Monsters.

You should be in no doubt that cannabis provides neither pleasure nor support. It does not help you relax. It does not make you more interesting or entertaining, nor does it help you enjoy a night out. It's not a reward, it's pure punishment – a highly addictive poison that destroys you physically and mentally.

You should also be clear that the only way to control cannabis consumption is not to take it. Cutting down or just having "the odd one" is not the best of both worlds, it's the worst of all worlds. As long as you put cannabis in your system, it will control you.

The only people who are not controlled by cannabis are people who don't take it – non-addicts. You become a non-addict the moment you stop taking cannabis without any desire to ever take it again. From that moment the Little Monster will begin to die. This is nothing to fear. On the contrary, you should rejoice in its death throes. Remember, it's your mortal enemy and it's leaving you for good.

The fear that has prevented you from escaping from the cannabis trap before now is the fear that you won't be able to enjoy or cope with life without cannabis. Non-addicts don't have this fear. Cannabis doesn't relieve the fear, it causes it. It's fantastic to be free of this fear.

A major cause of stress for some cannabis addicts is the effort they go to to keep their problem secret. It's much easier to overcome any problem if you're open and honest about it. But perhaps you find the idea of owning up unthinkable. You're afraid that your family and friends will be angry and will lose respect for you. It is possible that this will be the case. The people who love and trust you will be hurt, but in the end they will respect you for coming clean and will want to help.

It's more than likely, though, that the people you think you've been deceiving haven't been deceived at all. They will have noticed the change in your behaviour. They will already have been hurt by the change in your personality. They will have become suspicious of your inability to properly apply yourself to work and other commitments. The longer you go on trying to deceive them, the more these feelings will grow into distrust and alienation. Come clean and you give them the chance to understand why your behaviour has changed and to help you sort it out.

Don't be surprised to find that they're relieved by your admission. You may feel that your loved ones are not ready for the full story of your cannabis addiction and that "dumping it on them" would be unfair. That's ok. You're the best person to judge when the time is right to share the truth. Once you're enjoying the confidence and self-respect that comes with your newfound freedom, you'll be better equipped to work out the best way to come clean... if that's what you'd like to do.

On the other hand, you've most likely been completely open, or even brazen, about your cannabis use. If this is the case, those around you will not only notice the strange space between your lips where previously there was a seemingly never-ending spliff. They may also begin to notice some startling changes in your mood, behaviour, and demeanor. Enjoy those moments and don't allow yourself to be affected by people who are perhaps feeling unsettled by the change you have made.

When you find that you're enjoying life and coping with stress better as a non-dope addict, you'll no longer have to try to block your mind to the terrible effects that it had on you both physically and mentally. One of the huge bonuses of quitting is that you no longer need to worry about them.

It's time to kill the Little Monster and make your escape from the cannabis trap. If you feel the butterflies, that's perfectly natural. This is an exciting moment. Just remember, fear is not relieved by cannabis, it is caused by it.

You have nothing to fear from stopping, only marvellous gains to make. Think about the fly on the funnel of the pitcher plant. You could set it free by encouraging it to fly out while it still has a chance.

Remind yourself that cannabis does absolutely nothing for you whatsoever. It's a poison that causes immense damage to the length and quality of your life. You can stop the damage immediately by never taking it again. You have nothing to lose and everything to gain.

When you see a heroin addict, isn't it obvious to you that each time they inject the drug into a vein they're not curing their problem but making it worse? And the only thing that will end the problem for them is to stop taking heroin?

Think about the ex-con who's in danger of jeopardising his freedom by reoffending, because he's afraid of life outside prison. Put yourself in his position. Remind him of all the marvellous advantages there are to being free. Remind yourself of all the gains you will make without cannabis in your life.

- Better health
- Fewer mood swings
- Better relationships
- Higher self-esteem
- Less stress
- Better sleep
- Better concentration
- Clearer thinking
- More money
- More time

This is your chance to fly free. In fact, you can fly free any time you choose, so why wait? You have nothing to fear. Remember, dreadful things are guaranteed to happen as long as you stay in the cannabis trap. Escape and you can take control of putting your life back together.

You'll be amazed how good it feels to be free from the slavery of cannabis addiction.

Chapter 15

READY TO QUIT

The moment of your escape is marked by stubbing out your final joint and making a solemn vow never to take cannabis, or anything similar to it, again. If you haven't continued to take cannabis while you've been reading this book, that's not a problem, as long as you're confident that you've killed the Big Monster and you have no doubts whatsoever that you're not making a sacrifice or depriving yourself in any way. The vow, though, is important.

After you stop, you may be aware of the withdrawal for a few days. Remember this is not a physical pain, it's just the faint cries of the Little Monster wanting to be fed. However, light though it is, you should not ignore it. It's essential to keep in mind the fact that the Little Monster was created when you first started taking cannabis and it has continued to feed on every subsequent joint you've ever had.

As soon as you stop taking cannabis, you cut off the supply to the Little Monster and it begins to die. In its death throes it will try to entice you to feed it. Create a mental image of this parasite getting weaker and weaker and take pleasure in starving it to death. Keep this mental image with you at all times and make sure you don't respond to its death throes by thinking, "I need a joint."

Remember that the empty, insecure feeling was caused by your last joint. The feeling itself isn't pleasurable but you will enjoy it because you will understand the cause and know that the Little Monster inside you is dying. Noticing the Little Monster as it dies will make you smile and feel invincible rather than bother you.

Even if you do get that feeling of "I want a joint" for a few days, don't worry about it. Remember, it's not cannabis you want, it's relief from that nagging feeling, which will go away permanently provided you never take cannabis again.

If you were to have a joint, it would guarantee you suffer it for the rest of your life. It's just the Little Monster doing everything it can to tempt you to feed it. As long as you recognise that, you will find it easy to starve it to death. You now have complete control over it. It's no longer destroying you; you're destroying it and soon you will be free forever.

NO WAITING

Unlike the willpower method, with Easyway you don't have to wait for anything. You can start enjoying the genuine pleasure of being a non-dope addict from the moment you finish your final joint.

It takes just a few days for the physical withdrawal to pass. You may remember from personal experience that during this time, people who try to quit with the willpower method tend to feel completely obsessed with being denied what they see as their pleasure or support. Then, after about three weeks, there may come a moment when they suddenly realise that they haven't thought about cannabis for a while. It's an exciting feeling... and a dangerous moment.

They've gone from believing that life will always be miserable without being able to take cannabis, to believing that time will solve their problem. They feel great – surely this is the cure. It's time to celebrate. What possible harm could it do to reward themselves with just one joint?

The Big Monster is obviously still alive. They continue to believe that they've been denying themselves some sort of pleasure. If they're stupid enough to have a joint, they won't find it rewarding at all. It will give them no feeling of pleasure or support. Remember, the only reason they ever experienced the illusion of pleasure from cannabis is that it partially relieved the symptoms of withdrawal. But now that they're no longer withdrawing from cannabis, they will not even experience that illusion.

Nevertheless, that one joint is enough to revive the Little Monster.

Now panic starts to creep back in. They don't want their efforts to quit to be blown away so easily and for nothing, so they draw on their willpower and try not to give in to the urge to have another joint. But after a while the same thing happens. They regain their confidence and the temptation to have "just the one" rears its ugly head again. This time they can say to themselves, "I did it last time and didn't get hooked, so what's the harm in doing it again?"

Does this ring any bells? They're straying back into the trap.

Anyone who has tried to quit with the willpower method is likely to have experienced something similar. With Easyway, when you realise you haven't thought about cannabis for a while, your first thought is not to celebrate with a joint, it's:

GREAT – I'M FREE!

There is no feeling of deprivation. You can relax from the moment you finish your final joint and, rather than interpreting the feeling as "I want a joint", you think, '"Great! Isn't it marvellous! I don't ever have to go through that misery again."

Many ex-dope addicts who quit with the willpower method never get to the point where they can say that with certainty. They're never quite sure whether they've kicked it. The physical withdrawal symptoms feel like normal anxiety and stress, so when they experience these feelings they interpret them as "I want a joint".

Of course, taking cannabis at this stage wouldn't even give the illusion of relieving these natural pangs as they have no withdrawal, but they don't know that. They're still convinced that dope will help. The real stress is now increased because they believe that they're being deprived of a support that will ease the situation.

They're faced with a dilemma: go through the rest of their life believing they're missing out, or find out for sure. Sadly, the only way to do that is to take cannabis again. If they do, they find that their stress is not relieved – in fact, it's increased by their sense of disappointment at having given in to temptation. But they've revived the Little Monster and the outcome is that pretty soon they'll be taking dope just as before.

In a short while you'll have your final joint and make a solemn vow never to take cannabis, or anything similar, again. If this thought makes you panic, remind yourself of these simple facts:

• THE DRUGS INDUSTRY DEPENDS ON
THAT PANIC TO KEEP YOU HOOKED.

Have you ever thought about the havoc, the misery, the violence, the suffering that the cannabis industry inflicts across the world? We close our mind to it because it upsets us to think that we are fuelling all that crime and destruction. You don't need to turn your mind away from it anymore – you can feel fabulous to be free from it all.

• CANNABIS DOESN'T RELIEVE
THE PANIC, IT CAUSES IT.

Compose yourself. Do you really have any reason to panic? Nothing bad is going to happen as a result of you stopping. You have only marvellous gains to make.

Perhaps you're afraid of going into unknown territory. But there is nothing unknown about what you're about to do. It's something you've already done thousands of times before, every time you've finished your last joint at the end of the evening. This particular joint will be a very, very special one. It will be your last ever.

If you stopped taking cannabis before you started this book, you don't need to have a final joint – just confirm to yourself that you've already had one and then make the vow. Very soon you will feel stronger, both physically and mentally. You will have more energy, more confidence, more self-respect and more money. It's essential that you don't put off this wonderful freedom, not for a week, a day or a second.

Waiting for something to happen is one of the reasons why dope addicts using the willpower method find it so difficult. What are they waiting for? To find out if they'll ever take dope again? There's only one way to find that out...

So instead they're just left waiting, waiting, for the rest of their lives.

You become a non-dope addict the moment you finish your final joint and make the vow. What you're achieving is a new frame of mind, an understanding that cannabis does nothing for you and that by not taking it you're freeing yourself from a life of slavery, misery and degradation.

Replace any panic you may have felt with a feeling of excitement. You no longer need to feel ill, incapable, secretive or dishonest. You're about to discover the joy of taking control.

REJOICE!

This is going to be one of the best experiences of your life.

YOU'RE ABOUT TO BECOME FREE!

FINAL CHECKS

Earlier we compared the feeling of freedom you get when you escape the cannabis trap to the exhilaration of a parachute jump. What you're about to do will be one of the most exciting experiences of your life, so let's see that everything goes to plan and run through a final checklist to make sure you're properly prepared.

Your frame of mind should be, "Great! I don't need cannabis any more. I'm about to free myself from a prison of misery and degradation. I can't wait!"

You have every reason to celebrate. You're about to walk free from an evil trap, which has kept you imprisoned and severely disrupted your life, making you miserable, confused, frightened and angry. You're about to regain control over your life and banish those feelings of slavery and powerlessness for good. Very soon you will be a non-dope addict.

Take huge pride in your achievement; there are millions of dope addicts in the world who wish they could be in your shoes. Soon you'll rediscover the unbridled joy of feeling healthy, having nothing to hide, having time for the people you love and the things you love to do. While you were in the cannabis trap you forgot how to enjoy the genuine pleasures in life. You're about to get that major part of your life back.

YOUR NEW PERSPECTIVE

You've unravelled the brainwashing and dispelled the illusions that made you believe that cannabis gave you pleasure and support. You know and understand that cannabis is an addictive poison that will eventually destroy you, physically and mentally.

You have seen through the myths that kept you in the cannabis trap. You know that cannabis doesn't relieve stress and anxiety, it causes them; it's not a social lubricant, it's a social saboteur; it doesn't give you courage, it undermines it; and it doesn't help you think, it impairs judgement.

The reason you have not been able to stop taking cannabis in the past is not because there is something marvellous about it that you can't live without, nor is it a flaw in your personality. It's because you followed the wrong method. Now you understand that cannabis gives you neither pleasure nor support and the only reason you ever thought it did was because each joint brought a little bit of relief from the craving caused by the one before.

You have been addicted to a drug that takes control away from you but still tricks you into thinking you're in control. You have accepted that cannabis made you a slave and the only way to escape that slavery is to stop.

As you prepare for your final joint, you should be in no doubt that the decision you're taking isn't just the right one, it's the only one if you don't want to spend the rest of your life as a slave to cannabis. You should understand that any pangs you might feel after you stop are just the cries of the Little Monster as it breathes its last. Enjoy the feeling – it's the feeling of freedom. Nothing can take it away from you now. The only thing that might delay your escape is if you feel there might be a better time than now.

THE OPTIMUM TIME TO QUIT

Addicts tend to plan their attempts to quit to coincide with certain occasions. The two typical ones are a traumatic event, such as a health scare or a financial blow, and a "special" day, such as a birthday or New Year's Day. I call these "meaningless days", because they actually have no bearing whatsoever on your addiction, other than providing a target date for you to make your attempt to stop. That would be fine if it helped, but meaningless days actually cause more harm than good.

New Year's Day is the most popular of all meaningless days, being a clear marker of the end of one period and the beginning of another, a time for making resolutions. It also happens to have the lowest success rate.

The Christmas holidays are a time when we party more than usual and by New Year's Eve we're just about ready for a break. So we have one last binge and then, as the clock strikes midnight, we vow that we'll give the stuff a miss.

We very quickly start to feel cleansed, but the Little Monster is demanding its fix. If we're using the wrong method, we interpret these cries as "I want a joint" and though we may hold out to begin with, eventually the Big Monster will have its way and we find ourselves back in the trap.

Meaningless days only encourage us to go through the damaging cycle of half-hearted attempts to quit, bringing on the feeling of deprivation, followed by the sense of failure that reinforces the illusion that stopping is difficult and may be impossible. Dope addicts spend their lives looking for excuses to put off "the dreaded day". Meaningless days provide the perfect excuse to say, "I will quit, just not today."

Traumatic events tend to make us want to sort ourselves out in every way, including kicking those drugs. But these stressful times are also when your desire for the drug becomes strongest, because you regard it as a form of support. This is another ingenuity of the trap.

Some dope addicts choose their annual holiday, thinking that they'll be able to cope better away from the everyday stresses of work and home life and the usual temptations to take cannabis. Others pick a time when there are no social events coming up, where they will find it difficult not to take cannabis. These approaches might work for a while but they leave a lingering doubt: "OK, I've coped so far, but what about when I go back to work or that big party comes round?"

When you quit with Easyway, you should go out and handle stress and throw yourself into social occasions straight away, so that you can prove to yourself from the start that, even at times when you feared you would find it hard to get by without cannabis, you're still happy to be free.

So if you're trying to decide on the optimum time to make your break for freedom, consider this: if you saw someone you love hurting themselves repeatedly, what would you say? Would you ask them to stop the next time a convenient moment arises? Or would you ask them to stop at once?

DO IT NOW!

That's what the people who love you would say if they knew about your cannabis problem. You have everything you need to succeed. Like an athlete on the blocks at the start of the race, you're in peak condition to ensure success.

And if you just happen to be reading this now on a meaningless day or after a trauma, don't worry – with Easyway you will be successful regardless of the date, not because of it.

LET THE GOOD TIMES ROLL

Consider everything you stand to gain. Freedom from slavery, dishonesty, misery, anger, deceit, self-loathing, impotence – in short, your life back. No more scratching around for money; no more lying to people about what you need it for; no more hiding yourself away or trying to cover your tracks; no more self-loathing; no more feeling disappointed, guilty and weak.

Instead of all that misery you can look forward to living in the light, with your head held high, enjoying open, honest relationships, feeling in control of how you spend your time and money and finding joy in the genuine pleasures that you enjoyed before you walked into the cannabis trap.

With so much happiness to gain and so much misery to rid yourself of, what possible reason is there to wait? It's time for the seventh instruction:

MAKE A SOLEMN VOW NEVER TO TAKE CANNABIS, OR ANYTHING LIKE IT, AGAIN.

The vow you make marks the breaking point in the cycle of addiction. That's why it's important that you observe this ritual. As soon as you complete it, you're free.

And so the time has come. How do you feel?

You're about to escape from one of the most subtle and insidious traps ever devised. We've said all along that quitting is easy but that shouldn't diminish your sense of achievement. To follow the instructions, even when you may have doubted the outcome, to have gained a proper understanding of the nature of the trap – that requires considerable discipline and perseverance. It also takes courage.

So be proud of your achievement. You've reached a position that millions of dope addicts wish they could achieve. If you feel nervous, don't worry about it. That's completely normal at this stage and is no threat to your chances of success. When you make a parachute jump, the last-minute nerves quickly turn to exhilaration as your parachute opens and you realise that everything you've learned and prepared for is working exactly how they told you it would. This is the same.

It's impossible to put into words the utter joy of the person who has finally accepted that they don't need to take cannabis any more. The elation is incredible. It's like a huge, dark shadow being removed from your mind. You no longer need to despise yourself or have to worry about what the drug has been doing to your health, or all the money that you waste.

You no longer have to worry about where the next joint is coming from. You'll no longer feel weak, miserable, sordid, incomplete or guilty.

You're in that position now, standing by the plane door, ready to jump. You have all the knowledge and understanding you need to make this the best experience of your life. Soon you will be flying free. Remember:

YOU HAVE NOTHING TO FEAR.

The only thing that is facing sudden death is your cannabis addiction. You're not losing a friend; you have no reason to grieve. On the contrary, you should rejoice in the destruction of your mortal enemy.

Remind yourself that you're not "giving up" anything. You had no need to take cannabis before you started; you have no need to take cannabis now. Lifelong non-dope addicts and ex-dope addicts are quite happy without cannabis in their lives. What pleasure does it give? What support does it provide?

If you've followed and understood everything up to this point, you'll have come to the obvious conclusion:

CANNABIS HAS NO USEFUL PLACE IN YOUR LIFE.

Chapter 16

THE RITUAL OF
THE FINAL JOINT

Very soon you'll be asked to perform the ritual of the final joint. Before you do, it's essential that you're completely comfortable with the idea of never taking cannabis again. You must agree beyond any doubt that cannabis gives you no pleasure or support whatsoever and you're not making any sort of sacrifice.

You must be clear that the alternative to never having cannabis again is a lifetime of slavery and misery. It's a simple choice.

If you still feel as if you're being made to choose the lesser of two evils, ask yourself this: does it concern you that you might never suffer from flu again, or you might never suffer from a heart attack, or that you might never inject yourself with heroin? Presumably not. So why should it bother you that you will never again suffer the tyranny of dope addiction?

Cannabis addiction is a disease. It started when you began to consume the addictive poison. It ends with the ritual of the final joint.

If your mind is clear on these facts, you understand that there's nothing to "give up" and you follow all the instructions, quitting is ridiculously easy. You're doing it because you're sick of being a slave to dope and the difference between this time and previous times you've tried to quit is that instead of telling yourself, "I must never take cannabis again," you're thinking:

> **'GREAT! I NO LONGER HAVE TO WASTE MY TIME AND MONEY MAKING MYSELF MISERABLE AGAIN. I'M FREE!"**

This is a momentous occasion and one of the most important moves you'll ever make. You're freeing yourself from slavery and achieving something marvellous, something all cannabis addicts would love to achieve and something that everybody will admire and respect you for. Most importantly, you'll go right up in the estimations of one person in particular:

> **YOU.**

You should be feeling thrilled about ending the misery that cannabis has caused you after all this time. The thing that makes it difficult for people to quit with the willpower method is not the physical aggravation of withdrawal, it's the doubt, the uncertainty, the waiting to become a non-dope addict. With this method, you become a non-addict the moment you finish the ritual of your final joint and you make your vow never to take cannabis, or anything like it, again.

It's important to be able to make that vow with a feeling of venom, to visualise your triumph over the Little Monster and be able to say,

"YES! I'M A NON-DOPE ADDICT NOW. I'M FREE!"

Your mindset at this moment should be one of certainty. It's not enough to hope that you will never take cannabis again, you need to know. That said, don't worry if you feel apprehensive and nervous – there really isn't a right way or a wrong way to feel. So let's just go over the things that may cause you to doubt your decision.

First, consider this simple fact:

THERE IS ONLY ONE ESSENTIAL TO BEING A NON-DOPE ADDICT AND THAT IS NOT TO TAKE CANNABIS – EVER.

Then bring this to the front of your mind:

THERE IS ABSOLUTELY NOTHING TO GIVE UP.

In order to be a happy non-dope addict for life, it's essential never to have any desire for cannabis. If you have a desire to have just one puff, you'll have a desire to have another and another.

Get it clearly into your mind: it has to be all or nothing.

There are two other factors that can make you doubt your decision:

1. THE BELIEF THAT YOU HAVE AN ADDICTIVE PERSONALITY

Anyone can fall for the cannabis trap – and millions of people do. Even if you did have an addictive personality, that would simply mean that you easily get addicted, it wouldn't mean that you would find it difficult to stop.

2. OTHER DOPE ADDICTS

They're the ones who are losing out, not you. Having read this book, you have infinitely more expertise on the subject of drug addiction than they have. Pity them if you like but do not envy them. They're still in the trap, you are escaping.

You're about to make the decision to end your cannabis taking and vow never to have it again. If you made that decision before you started reading this book, you just need to reconfirm the decision in your mind now. This is the moment when you walk free.

Think about the misery and suffering that cannabis has caused you. Visualise the Little Monster and how it has dominated your life. Imagine it laughing at you. This is the time for your revenge. Make your vow. No more slavery! No more misery! You're cutting off its lifeline and destroying that evil tyrant once and for all.

I WOULD NOW LIKE YOU TO HAVE YOUR FINAL JOINT PLEASE.

If you haven't already stopped, now is the time to have your final joint.

Take a moment.

Now think about what you've achieved. You will never do that again.

REJOICE! YOU'RE FREE!

Now make your vow: promise yourself that you will never take cannabis, or anything similar, again.

SEAL THE DEAL

You've achieved something incredible – possibly the most important achievement of your life. Revel in your victory. You want this moment to stick in your mind.

Right now you're fired up with powerful reasons to stop, but as the days, weeks and years go by, the memory of how you were feeling about cannabis today will probably dim. So fix those thoughts in your mind now while they're vivid, so that even if your memory of the details should diminish, your resolution never to take cannabis again does not.

You can easily guard against any moments of doubt in the future by planning for them now. In a few months you'll find it hard to believe that you once found it necessary to take cannabis, let alone how it controlled your life. You may also lose your fear of getting hooked again. Be aware now, in advance, that this can be a danger. You might have moments when you're on a complete natural high, surrounded by people on dope, or you might suffer a trauma and your guard will be down. Prepare yourself for these situations now and make it part of your vow that, if and when they come, there is no way that you'll be led into starting to take cannabis again.

Be clear in your mind that cannabis neither made the good times better nor relieved stress during the bad times. It did the complete opposite.

Now you're ready to move on. You don't have to wait for anything. Embrace this moment with a feeling of excitement and elation. You've freed yourself from the bonds of addiction.

THE WHOLE SORDID NIGHTMARE IS OVER.

Chapter 17

ENJOY FREEDOM

Congratulations! You've done it! You're now a non-dope addict and will remain one for the rest of your life, provided you never lose faith in your decision. You can immediately get on with enjoying the many pleasures that life has to offer.

For a few days, you may detect the cries of the Little Monster as it goes through its death throes. This is nothing to worry about, so don't try to block it from your mind. Recognise the cries and rejoice in what they signify – the death of the monster that has held you enslaved for all this time.

As a cannabis addict you felt compelled to feed the Little Monster. Now you don't have to do anything. That's the method for killing the Little Monster:

DO NOTHING.

It's that easy.

Prepare your response to the dying cries of the Little Monster. Instead of thinking, "I want a joint but I'm not allowed one," think, "This is the Little Monster demanding its fix. This is what dope addicts suffer throughout their addicted lives. Non-dope addicts don't suffer this feeling. Isn't it great?! I'm a non-dope addict and I'm free!"

Focus on the feeling and notice that there is no physical pain. Any discomfort you might feel is not because you've stopped taking dope but because you started in the first place. Be absolutely clear that having another joint, far from relieving that discomfort, would only ensure that you suffered it for the rest of your life.

Prepare your mind to respond in this way and any withdrawal pangs will become moments of pleasure. Rejoice in the Little Monster's death throes and feel no guilt about it. After all, it's been killing you, making you miserable and keeping you a slave for too long.

Consign your previous attempts to quit to history. The willpower method leaves people forever moping for something they hope they'll never do, forever waiting for nothing to happen. But when you have no desire to take cannabis, you don't have to wait or mope for anything. You don't have to stand by and grit your teeth while the Little Monster dies, you can get straight on with enjoying life.

THE RETURN OF GENUINE PLEASURES

One of the great benefits of becoming free from cannabis is that you rediscover how to enjoy life's genuine pleasures. When you're addicted to the drug you lose the ability fully to enjoy the things that you used to enjoy before you became hooked – the things that non-addicts enjoy most: reading books, getting out and about, watching entertainment, social occasions, exercise, sex. Now that you're free from dope, you have all these pleasures to get excited about again.

Situations you have come to regard as unstimulating, or even irritating, will become enjoyable again: simple things like spending time with your loved ones, going for walks, chatting to friends. Work will become more enjoyable, as you find you're better able to engage with it and concentrate, to think creatively and to handle stress.

At the same time, you'll become more clear-sighted about the things you don't like doing. Most people suddenly realise when they stop taking cannabis that they've wasted a lot of time going to boring events that gave them no pleasure at all. It's just another way that cannabis steals excitement, ambition and energy in all aspects of life.

Deciding to stop doing things that you find dull and boring is incredibly empowering. When you cut cannabis out of your life, you regain the ability to see things as they really are and make better decisions about how you fill your time.

BAD DAYS

Everyone has bad days from time to time. Be prepared for them. They have nothing to do with the fact that you're no longer on cannabis. The only connection is that when you stop taking the drug you find the bad days don't come around so frequently and when they do, you feel better equipped to cope with them.

You might well find that when you have bad days, or even very good days, the thought of taking dope does enter your mind. That's not unusual and it's nothing to worry about. You don't have to push the thought out of your mind, you just have to recognise it for what it is: a remnant from the days when you responded to every setback or celebration by using cannabis.

It doesn't mean you're still vulnerable to the trap, it just means you're still adjusting to your newfound freedom. You can dismiss the thought very quickly by thinking, "Great! I don't have to use cannabis any more. I'm free!"

There are just a few final instructions to see you through your life as a non-dope addict. The eighth instruction is one you should already be clear about:

NEVER DOUBT YOUR DECISION TO QUIT.

It's essential that you never doubt or question your decision to stop. Never make the mistake that people on the willpower method make, of craving the drug again. If you do you'll put yourself in the same impossible position as them: miserable if you don't and even more miserable if you do.

The ninth instruction is:

IGNORE ANYTHING YOU READ ABOUT CANNABIS, OR HEAR ABOUT CANNABIS, THAT CONFLICTS WITH EASYWAY.

Much of what you've read in this book will have been new to you. You were required to open your mind but now you can see the logic in it. Be sceptical about anything that contradicts what you've read here and you'll be happily immune to it.

The tenth and final instruction is one that you have already decided for yourself:

NEVER TAKE CANNABIS AGAIN.

And that's it. You've done it! Never forget that if you ever have any uncertainties or concerns about cannabis, or a question arises in your mind, or you just have a nagging doubt about your freedom – everyone at Easyway is here for you. We answer hundreds and thousands of questions a year and never tire of doing so…supporting former addicts in their enjoyment of their freedom makes us incredibly happy – so please don't hesitate to get in touch.

All that is left for me to say is CONGRATULATIONS on being free and all the best for your future:

FREE FROM CANNABIS!

ALLEN CARR'S
EASYWAY CENTRES

The following list indicates the countries where Allen Carr's Easyway To Stop Smoking Centres are currently operational.

Check www.allencarr.com for the latest additions to this list.

The success rate at the centres, based on the three-month money-back guarantee, is over 90 per cent.

Selected centres also offer sessions that deal with alcohol, other drugs and weight issues. Please check with your nearest centre, listed below, for details.

Allen Carr's Easyway guarantee that you will find it easy to stop at the centres or your money back.

JOIN US!

Allen Carr's Easyway Centres have spread throughout the world with incredible speed and success. Our global franchise network now covers more than 150 cities in over 45 countries. This amazing growth has been achieved entirely organically. Former addicts, just like you, were so impressed by the ease with which they stopped that they felt inspired to contact us to see how they could bring the method to their region.

If you feel the same, contact us for details on how to become an Allen Carr's Easyway To Stop Smoking or an Allen Carr's Easyway To Stop Drinking franchisee.

Email us at: join-us@allencarr.com including your full name, postal address and region of interest.

SUPPORT US!

No, don't send us money!

You have achieved something really marvellous. Every time we hear of someone escaping from the sinking ship, we get a feeling of enormous satisfaction.

It would give us great pleasure to hear that you have freed yourself from the slavery of addiction, so please visit the following web page where you can tell us of your success, inspire others to follow in your footsteps and hear about ways you can help to spread the word.

 www.allencarr.com/fanzone

You can "like" our Facebook page here **www.facebook.com/ AllenCarr**

Together, we can help further Allen Carr's mission: to cure the world of addiction.

CENTRES

Allen Carr's Easyway
Worldwide Head Office
Park House, 14 Pepys Road, Raynes Park
London SW20 8NH
Tel: +44 (0) 208 944 7761
Email: mail@allencarr.com
Website: www.allencarr.com

Worldwide Press Office
Tel: +44 (0) 7970 88 44 52
Email: Media@allencarr.com

UK Centre and Central Booking Line
0800 389 2115 (Freephone)

United Kingdom
Australia
Austria
Belgium
Brazil
Bulgaria
Canada
Chile
Colombia
Cyprus
Czech Republic
Denmark
Estonia
Finland
France
Germany
Greece
Guatemala
Hong Kong
Hungary
Iceland
India
Iran
Israel
Italy
Japan

Lithuania
Mauritius
Mexico
Netherlands
New Zealand
Norway
Peru
Poland
Portugal
Republic of Ireland
Romania
Russia
Saudi Arabia
Serbia
Singapore
Slovenia
South Africa
South Korea
Spain
Sweden
Switzerland
Turkey
Ukraine
UAE
USA

OTHER ALLEN CARR PUBLICATIONS

Allen Carr's revolutionary Easyway method is available in a wide variety of formats, including digitally as audiobooks and ebooks, and has been successfully applied to a broad range of subjects.

For more information about Easyway publications, please visit **shop.allencarr.com**